Accession no.
36230228

Rapid Mental Health Nursing

D1375340

Rapid Mental Health Nursing

Grahame Smith
Principal Lecturer and Subject Head (Allied Health)
Liverpool John Moores University
Liverpool

Rebecca Rylance
Senior Lecturer in Mental Health Nursing
Liverpool John Moores University
Liverpool

LIS - LIBRARY

Date	Fund
24/5/18	nm—War
Order No.	
2874222.	
University of Chester	

WILEY Blackwell

This edition first published 2016 © 2016 by John Wiley and Sons, Ltd

Registered Office
John Wiley & Sons, Ltd, The Atrium, Southern Gate, Chichester, West Sussex, PO19 8SQ, UK

Editorial Offices
9600 Garsington Road, Oxford, OX4 2DQ, UK
The Atrium, Southern Gate, Chichester, West Sussex, PO19 8SQ, UK
111 River Street, Hoboken, NJ 07030-5774, USA

For details of our global editorial offices, for customer services and for information about how to apply for permission to reuse the copyright material in this book please see our website at www.wiley.com/wiley-blackwell.

The right of the author to be identified as the author of this work has been asserted in accordance with the UK Copyright, Designs and Patents Act 1988.

All rights reserved. No part of this publication may be reproduced, stored in a retrieval system, or transmitted, in any form or by any means, electronic, mechanical, photocopying, recording or otherwise, except as permitted by the UK Copyright, Designs and Patents Act 1988, without the prior permission of the publisher.

Designations used by companies to distinguish their products are often claimed as trademarks. All brand names and product names used in this book are trade names, service marks, trademarks or registered trademarks of their respective owners. The publisher is not associated with any product or vendor mentioned in this book. It is sold on the understanding that the publisher is not engaged in rendering professional services. If professional advice or other expert assistance is required, the services of a competent professional should be sought.

The contents of this work are intended to further general scientific research, understanding, and discussion only and are not intended and should not be relied upon as recommending or promoting a specific method, diagnosis, or treatment by health science practitioners for any particular patient. The publisher and the author make no representations or warranties with respect to the accuracy or completeness of the contents of this work and specifically disclaim all warranties, including without limitation any implied warranties of fitness for a particular purpose. In view of ongoing research, equipment modifications, changes in governmental regulations, and the constant flow of information relating to the use of medicines, equipment, and devices, the reader is urged to review and evaluate the information provided in the package insert or instructions for each medicine, equipment, or device for, among other things, any changes in the instructions or indication of usage and for added warnings and precautions. Readers should consult with a specialist where appropriate. The fact that an organization or Website is referred to in this work as a citation and/or a potential source of further information does not mean that the author or the publisher endorses the information the organization or Website may provide or recommendations it may make. Further, readers should be aware that Internet Websites listed in this work may have changed or disappeared between when this work was written and when it is read. No warranty may be created or extended by any promotional statements for this work. Neither the publisher nor the author shall be liable for any damages arising herefrom.

Library of Congress Cataloging-in-Publication Data

Names: Smith, Grahame, author. | Rylance, Rebecca, 1969– , author.
Title: Rapid mental health nursing / Grahame Smith, Rebecca Rylance.
Description: Chichester, West Sussex ; Hoboken, NJ : John Wiley & Sons Inc., 2016. |
    Includes bibliographical references and index.
Identifiers: LCCN 2015042381 | ISBN 9781119045007 (pbk.)
Subjects: | MESH: Mental Disorders–nursing–Problems and Exercises. |
    Psychiatric Nursing–methods–Problems and Exercises.
Classification: LCC RC440 | NLM WY 18.2 | DDC 616.89/0231–dc23
LC record available at http://lccn.loc.gov/2015042381

A catalogue record for this book is available from the British Library.

Wiley also publishes its books in a variety of electronic formats. Some content that appears in print may not be available in electronic books.

Cover image: ©Alina Vincent Photography, LLC/Getty Images.

Set in 9.5/11.5pt Frutiger by SPi Global, Pondicherry, India
Printed and bound in Malaysia by Vivar Printing Sdn Bhd

1 2016

Contents

Conditions

Specific issues

Introduction

This book complements *Mental Health Nursing at a Glance* and, similar to that text, is written with the pre-registration mental health nursing student in mind as a 'revision or notes' text; it is also designed to be a refresher text for registered mental health nurses. The structure of each chapter is intended to support the UK student's learning journey; each chapter is explicitly underpinned by the Nursing & Midwifery Council's (NMC's) *Standards for Pre-registration Nursing Education* (NMC 2010). As befits a *Rapid* series text, each chapter is a concise summary of the subject being explored and, in addition, this book has been designed to be easy for the mental health nursing student to carry around.

To place the book within a professional context, the NMC's Standards for Pre-registration Nursing Education aim to:

> …. enable nurses to give and support high-quality care in rapidly changing environments. They reflect how future services are likely to be delivered, acknowledge future public health priorities and address the challenges of long-term conditions, an aging population, and providing more care outside hospitals. Nurses must be equipped to lead, delegate, supervise and challenge other nurses and healthcare professionals. They must be able to develop practice, and promote and sustain change. As graduates they must be able to think analytically, use problem-solving approaches and evidence in decision-making, keep up with technical advances and meet future expectations.
>
> (NMC 2010: 4–5)

Further to this aim, the NMC expect that by the end of training a pre-registration nursing student will be competent and possess the required knowledge, skills and attitudes. These requirements are set out in a competency framework for each field of nursing, which is organised into four domains:

- professional values;
- communication and interpersonal skills;
- nursing practice and decision-making;
- leadership, management and team working.

Each domain describes the competencies the student is expected to achieve by end of their training, and each chapter of this book is underpinned by these domain competencies. In addition to generic skills, mental health nursing students are expected to develop field-specific skills. These different skill types complement each other to ensure that, at the point of registration, a mental health nurse has a holistic set of competencies that they can apply in many different contexts. Taking the different skill types into consideration, the first section of this book is focused on generic skills, followed by two field-specific sections. Overall the book is divided into three main sections:

- Essential skills and knowledge;
- Conditions;
- Specific issues.

These three main sections are supported by:

- Appendixes, including essential anatomy and physiology, clinical procedures;
- Revision questions;
- Glossary;
- References, further reading and useful resources.

The structure of the book will provide the student nurse with a clear sense of direction in their journey towards qualification. It is, however, not a replacement for more in-depth texts within the field of mental health nursing. In addition, the student nurse should apply both generic and field competencies in an integrated and fluid way, and with the support of their mentor.

Essential skills and knowledge

Rapid Mental Health Nursing, First Edition. Grahame Smith and Rebecca Rylance.
© 2016 John Wiley & Sons, Ltd. Published 2016 by John Wiley & Sons, Ltd.

Assessment

Background

Assessment is a fundamental part of mental health nursing practice; it establishes an understanding of the service user's situation through a process of asking questions. Assessment is not a one-off, it is an ongoing process which is built on partnership working, starting with a service user's admission to mental health services and continuing until they are discharged. Information gathered from the initial assessment process is the first step in planning and delivering care across services to ensure that the care delivered is effective and based upon the service user's needs.

Assessment can be broadly divided into two categories or methods:

- formal assessment, including checklists, questionnaires, rating scales, tools, and structured interviews;
- informal assessment, when information is collected through less formal and planned methods, such as day-to-day observations and interactions.

Both methods provide the mental health nurse with valuable information, and both methods should have equal weight; however, formal assessment tends to be viewed as more objective and value-free. Sometimes this can lead to information gathered through formal assessment methods having more weight than informally gathered information. The strength of using both methods is that information can be triangulated in way that captures the whole clinical picture rather than just part of the picture.

Assessment information should describe the service user's situation, both generally and specifically; it should also identify the degree to which any identified problem has impacted, and is impacting upon, the service user's ability to function. To elicit this information the nurse should use:

- open questions to scope the broad issues;
- more probing questions to identify the specific issues;
- closed questions to confirm their understanding of the specific issues is correct.

Professional skills

Mental health nurses should be able to:

- undertake nursing assessments that are comprehensive, systematic and holistic;
- utilise assessment information to plan, deliver and evaluate care;
- work in partnership with the service user, their carers and their families throughout the assessment to negotiate goals and develop a personalised plan of care.

Types of assessment

Mental health nursing assessments should be holistic and, as such, during the assessment process the nurse should gather a wide range of information about the following:

- physical health and functioning;
- psychological functioning;
- social functioning;
- spiritual needs.

A variety of assessment tools should be used to gather specific information about:

- risk;
- history;
- symptoms;
- social functioning;
- quality of life.

Assessment tools

Specific assessment tools used in mental health nursing include:

- Brief Psychiatric Rating Scale (http://www.public-health.uiowa.edu/icmha/outreach/documents/bprs_expanded.pdf);
- Beck Depression Inventory (http://mhinnovation.net/sites/default/files/downloads/innovation/research/bdi%20with%20interpretation.pdf);
- Positive and Negative Syndrome Scale (http://egret.psychol.cam.ac.uk/medicine/scales/panss.pdf);
- Beliefs About Voices Questionnaire (http://www.hearingvoices.org.uk/pdf/bavqr.pdf);
- Rosenberg Self-Esteem Scale (http://www.yorku.ca/rokada/psyctest/rosenbrg.pdf);
- Health of the Nation Outcome Scales (http://amhocn.org/static/files/assets/2ad72217/honos_glossary.pdf);
- Camberwell Assessment of Need (http://www.researchintorecovery.com/files/cansas-p.pdf);
- Social Functioning Scale (https://mh4ot.files.wordpress.com/2012/05/social-functioning-scale.pdf);
- Quality of Life Scale (http://www.mentalhealth.com/qol/imhqolscale.pdf);
- Patient Health Questionnaire (http://phqscreeners.com/pdfs/02_phq-9/english.pdf).

Assessment skills

The therapeutic relationship should drive the assessment process which should be person centred, collaborative and underpinned by the use of effective communication skills such as questioning, active listening, clarifying and summarising. The skills required of mental health nurses are to:

- interview — ask questions about behaviours and symptoms;
- observe — record what they see;
- measure — rate the severity of behaviours and symptoms.

Mental health nurses should utilise all three strategies. It is also important to focus on what the service user can do rather than what they cannot do; this strengths-based approach underpins the recovery process.

Assessment and care delivery

Assessment information is used to inform the delivery of care. It assists the mental health nurse and the service user in partnership to identify what the issues are and what needs to be addressed. The next step after assessment is to consider what the partnership is trying to achieve, and what change the partnership would like to take place and by when. After this step the partnership can consider what interventions would be the most useful, and it is at this stage that the relevant clinical guidelines need to be taken into consideration. The final step is to review the process — were the goals achieved? If not why not? Is there another approach that could be considered? Overall the process should look like this:

1. assessment;
2. care planning and goal setting;
3. care delivery;
4. evaluation.

Care planning

Background

Care planning follows on from the previous section on assessment. Care planning is concerned with the practice of planning care with a service user in order to meet their individual health and well-being needs. Traditionally, a nurse would assess a service user's needs, identify their problems, plan care and evaluate the success of the plan. However, there has recently been a significant shift within mental health services to refocus the clinical language to that of goal identification instead of problem identification. When goals have been identified (utilising a strength-based approach) a collaborative plan of care is developed to help the service user achieve their goals. Regular evaluation, preferably with the service user and their family as well as the clinical team, will ensure that the care plan is effective and also responsive to any changes.

The Care Programme Approach (CPA; The Care Programme Approach Association 2008) is the key framework which informs the care-planning process in mental health in the UK. The CPA aims to ensure that people have access to services to meet their diverse needs, choices and preferences. Only through collaboration with the service user, their carer, the CPA coordinator, and health and social care professionals can an appropriate plan of care be devised. A useful document that describes effective collaboration is *Ten Essential Shared Capabilities* (DoH 2004), which lists the key principles for inclusive practice for nurses across health and community settings:

- working in partnership;
- respecting diversity;
- practising ethically;
- challenging inequality;
- promoting recovery;
- identifying needs and strengths;
- providing service-user-centred care;
- making a difference;
- promoting safety and positive risk taking;
- personal development and learning.

Professional skills
Mental health nurses should:

- actively empower service users and carers to be involved in the care-planning process;
- understand the public health dimension of planning and delivering care;
- ensure a service users physical, social, economic, psychological and spiritual needs are addressed when planning and delivering care;
- ensure that care planning and delivery is person centred, collaborative, evidence-based and framed by the relevant ethical and legal frameworks.

Partnership
It is vital that nurses work in partnership with people experiencing mental health issues and empower them to make decisions about their care. By utilising a recovery-focused approach, nurses can support a service user to achieve well-being and recovery. Therefore, it is important for mental health nurses to assess each service user's needs holistically, facilitate goal setting, devise a care plan collaboratively and then evaluate it regularly. In the UK, the NMC's professional code of conduct (Nursing & Midwifery Council 2015) is central to the nursing process.

Nursing models
The body of knowledge for nursing is supported by a number of nursing models that are highly abstract and broad in nature; however

they provide a structured way to make sense of the care planning and care-delivery process. Nursing knowledge can be categorised in the following four ways (Carper 1978):

- empiric — explaining and predicting;
- aesthetic — particular and unique to the situation;
- personal — interpersonal;
- ethical — doing the right thing.

The following is a list of the most well-known nursing models:

- Henderson's nursing model;
- Johnson's behavioural system model;
- King's open systems model;
- Neuman's systems model;
- Nightingale's nursing theory;
- Orem's self-care model;
- Peplau's interpersonal relations model;
- Rogers science of unitary human beings;
- Roper's activities of living model;
- Roy's adaptation model.

Peplau's interpersonal relations model (Peplau 1952) is specific to mental health nursing and articulates the view that mental health nursing is an interpersonal and therapeutic process. Nursing models are applied to practice through a framework that provides a systematic process; in the case of Peplau's model, the Tidal Model of mental health recovery provides this framework. It is important to note that mental health nursing is also heavily influenced by biological theories, psychodynamic theories, learning theories, cognitive theories and social theories.

Discharge planning and the CPA

The CPA provides:

- a systematic assessment of needs and risk;
- a care-planning process that is based on needs and risk;
- a care coordinator;
- regular reviews.

The CPA influences the discharge planning process in two ways. Firstly, a mental health service user discharged from inpatient services, where supported by community mental health services, is likely to be placed on a CPA plan. Secondly, the service user being supported by community services is discharged from the CPA when it is deemed by those services that they are well enough.

Clinical decision-making

Background

Mental health nurses are organisationally and professionally accountable for their day-to-day clinical decisions. Some decisions are more complex than others, but irrespective of their complexity the nurse needs to be able to justify the decisions they make. Therefore clinical decisions should be based on evidence, and the nurse should be able to explain which evidence they used and why. The motivation behind the use of evidence should not be to defend a decision, rather the use of evidence should be a regular part of the clinical decision-making process, which actively involves other professionals and, more importantly, service users and carers.

When delivering care mental health nurses have to be effective decision makers. This need for effective clinical decision-making is driven by an expectation that care delivery is of a high standard, and nurses are publically accountable for the clinical decisions they make. To make a clinical decision the mental health nurse needs to:

- identify the issue/s;
- analyse the evidence;
- consider the options;
- plan a way forward;
- implement the decision;
- evaluate the outcome.

Making a decision in this way can appear logical and unemotional, and it is important to note that decision-making in clinical practice will, most of the time, have an emotional context. That is why the evaluation of the decision is so vital and should be linked into the nurse's reflective practices, such as clinical supervision. As there is a values-based context to mental health nursing there is also a need to be ethically sensitive and pay attention to the service user's viewpoint, especially when dealing with the sensitive issue of restricting a service user's freedoms.

Professional skills

Mental health nurses should:

- ensure that clinical decision-making is person centred and evidence based, and the outcomes of the decision-making process are evaluated;
- make decisions in partnership with others involved in the care process to ensure high-quality care;
- signpost to others when the complexity of clinical decisions requires specialist knowledge and expertise;
- recognise and address the ethical context of clinical decision-making in a way that focuses on agreed and acceptable solutions.

Risk

Decision-making has an element of risk; which the best option? In the mental health field practitioners can become defensive, especially when dealing with harms, and this might mean that a decision is more inclined towards being risk adverse, which might not be in best interest of the service user. To make a considered decision the nurse has to weigh up all potential outcomes and also factor in the needs and wants of the service user.

Analysing the evidence

Analysing and using the best evidence is a key part of the clinical decision-making process. The focus of this approach is to provide the best care available. Using the best evidence ensures that established care delivery is also supported by research-based evidence; the evidence used in this approach is usually scientific evidence. Utilising evidence-based knowledge in the clinical decision-making process requires the mental health nurse to be able to:

- identify the clinical issue;
- understand the issue as a clinical question;
- search the scientific literature;
- critique different types of evidence;
- deliver the chosen intervention;
- evaluate the delivery of the intervention.

In addition to choosing a specific intervention, the mental health nurse will also have to consider whether this intervention can be situated within the therapeutic relationship in a way that reflects the specific needs of the mental health service user.

Challenges

Decisions are not made in isolation and there are a number of influencing factors that the mental health nurse will have to take into consideration, including:

- Is there enough information available to make an effective decision?
- What are the timescales?
- What are we trying to achieve?
- Are the required skills and resources available to implement the chosen intervention?
- What are the risks of either taking action or not taking action?

Real-time decisions

Systematic approaches to decision-making can be useful, but it has to be accepted that a number of clinical decisions have to be made in real time. For example, a mental health service user may be actively seeking to harm themselves; in this situation the mental health nurse will need to act quickly and keep the service user safe. Acting quickly is not an excuse for not doing the right thing, however, and the mental health nurse will need to ensure that they are properly prepared to be able to deal with this type of situation effectively. Being properly prepared stems from:

- having a good foundation of knowledge and skills;
- being able to utilise different forms of knowledge such as empiric, aesthetic, personal and ethical knowledge;
- having the commitment to engage in reflective practice that is structured and protected;
- working in true partnership with mental health service users;
- being a lifelong learner.

Clinical observations

Background

A key role of mental health nurses is to develop a comprehensive and personalised plan of care, and this plan of care should consider a service user's physical health needs. To ensure that a service user's physical needs are systematically assessed the mental health nurse will need to undertake a number of clinical observations.

Undertaking clinical observations is an important, but sometimes forgotten, part of the mental health nurse's role. This is particularly the case when you consider that mental health service users have higher rate of physical health needs than the general (DoH 2011a). For data from clinical observations to be meaningful in the long term they need to be integrated with information obtained from other sources, such as clinical examination and medical history data. In the short-term, however, clinical observations (also known as vital signs) can assist in the process of determining whether the nurse is dealing with a physical emergency. Clinical observations include:

- temperature;
- pulse rate;
- respiratory rate;
- blood pressure;
- peak flow rate;
- urinalysis;
- blood glucose level;
- central venous pressure;
- neurological observations.

Clinical observations are sometimes called vital signs and historically consist of temperature, pulse rate, respiratory rate and blood pressure. In addition to these vital signs mental health nurses also need to be familiar with observations of peak flow rate, urinalysis and blood glucose level.

Professional skills

Mental health nurses should be able to:

- collect and interpret routine data related to the care-planning process;
- measure and record a services user's weight, height, temperature, pulse rate, respiratory rate and blood pressure;
- respond appropriately when a service user's vital signs are outside the normal range or when there is a sudden deterioration in service user's vital signs;
- carry out and interpret routine diagnostic tests, such as a urinalysis.

Temperature

Normal body temperature is in the range 36.0–37.2°C. Body temperature should be monitored in case it is too high (a body temperature above 37.5°C is called pyrexia) or too low (a body temperature below 35.0°C is called hypothermia). Temperature readings can be taken by digital or non-digital thermometers at the mouth, forehead, ear canal or under the arm.

Pulse rate

Measuring the pulse rate gives an indication of how well the heart is functioning; counting the pulse or beats per minute is equivalent to measuring heart rate. A 'normal' pulse rate for a healthy adult is between 60 and 100 beats per minute. The pulse can be felt in any place where an artery can be compressed against a bone, such as the neck, wrist, knee, inside of the elbow and near the ankle joint. The pulse is usually taken at the wrist — the radial site — and not only is the rate noted but also the rhythm and amplitude (pulse strength).

Respiratory rate

The role of the respiratory system is to ensure that the body has enough oxygen to function correctly and toxic carbon dioxide is removed; the respiratory process consists of:

- ventilation — movement of air in and out of the lungs;
- external respiration — gas exchange;
- transport — movement of respiratory gases;
- internal respiration — delivery of oxygen and uptake of carbon dioxide.

Generally, a respiratory assessment consists of assessing the:

- airway — checking for obstructions;
- breathing — rate, rhythm and depth;
- skin colour — looking for cyanosis (a blue tone to the skin);
- use of accessory muscles — such as breathing through flared nostrils or pursed lips;
- general condition — level of consciousness.

Blood pressure

Blood pressure is a measure of the force of blood against the vessel walls such as the brachial artery in the upper arm, which is the usual site for measuring blood pressure. Blood pressure as a value is expressed as systolic pressure over diastolic pressure; systolic pressure is a measure of the peak pressure of the left ventricle in the heart and diastolic pressure is a measure of aortic pressure at its lowest. Normal blood pressure, which is measured in millimetres of mercury (mmHg), can range from 110 to 140 mmHg for systolic pressure, and from 70 to 80 mmHg for diastolic pressure. When an individual's sustained blood pressure is greater than 140/90 mmHg this is defined as hypertension; if they have a systolic reading less than 100 mmHg this is defined as hypotension.

Clinical risk in mental health

Background

The focus of this chapter is on managing risk within a specific context; where there is the potential that a mental health service user poses a risk to self and/or others, or is at risk from others, including neglect. Risk management in this context needs to be in partnership with the service user; it also needs to be systematic. The process of managing risk is dynamic in nature as levels of risk can change quite quickly. At times the management of risk can be perceived as controlling to the service user especially where risk is managed through the use of legally restricting a service user's freedoms.

Managing clinical risk within mental health care involves calculating the likelihood that harms, or the threat of harms, will occur. To manage this potential risk the mental health nurse will undertake an assessment of risk; any risks identified will be documented and communicated appropriately to the multidisciplinary team. The next stage is to manage risk systematically through the implementation of a risk-management plan.

Professional skills

Mental health nurses should:

- recognise and manage risk in a way that is person centred and recovery focused, and protects vulnerable individuals;
- empower choices and promote well-being while managing risk;
- work positively and proactively with individuals who are at risk using evidence-based models of care that prevent, reduce and minimise risk;
- manage risk both independently and as part of a team approach in a way that promotes effective communication, positive risk management and continuity of care across services.

Risk assessment

Managing risk within the field of mental health has been influenced by a number of governmental initiatives and policies in the UK, one of these being the Care Programme Approach (CPA; CPAA 2008). Based upon this approach when assessing risk the mental health nurse should consider:

- What is the type of risk; for example, self-harm or neglect? To others or from others?
- How recently did the risk-related incidents occur? How severe is the risk and what is the level of intent?
- How frequently have the risk-related incidents occurred?
- When do the risk-related incidents happen? Are there trigger factors? Is the individual under the influence of drugs and/or alcohol when the risk-related incidents occur?
- What is the service user's understanding of the identified risks? What is their present mental state and do they have mental capacity?

Types of risk assessment

Risk-assessment approaches include:

- unstructured risk assessment — clinical risk information is accrued unsystematically;
- actuarial risk assessment — risk information is collected and processed using a risk-assessment tool and a risk score is calculated;
- structured risk assessment — evidence-based research influences the types of risk information collected, usually through the use of specific risk-assessment tools. This information is then discussed in combination with both the nurse's knowledge of the service user and the service user's own views.

A structured approach is generally thought to be best practice; however, this is dependent upon the skill of the nurse and the availability of suitable risk-assessment tools.

Managing risk

Managing risk should be based on a positive risk-management approach with a focus on collaboration and recovery especially when engaging in supportive observations of service users at risk. The level of supportive observation is implemented as indicated by the level of identified risk:

- level 1 (general) observation: the minimum level of observation for all inpatients;
- level 2 (intermittent) observation: the service-user's location on the ward is checked every 15–30 minutes;
- level 3 observation: the service user is kept within sight at all times;
- level 4 observation: the service user is kept within an arm's-length of the observing nurse.

Using a positive and supportive approach prevents over-defensive practice and promotes therapeutic engagement, a positive approach includes:

- actively listening to the service user's views;
- collaborative action planning and decision-making;
- thoughtful consideration of potential benefits and harms when deciding on actions;
- implementing decisions that involve an element of risk where the benefits outweigh the risk;
- ensuring that the risk-management plan is fully communicated.

When managing risk it is useful to note that risks can be static or dynamic. Static risks are risk-related incidents that happened in the past, or factors such as age or employment that indicate that an individual is statistically at risk. Dynamic risks are factors that influence risk constantly, such as an individual's mental state or their social circumstances. By taking into account the dynamic nature of risk and how it might change over time, the nurse can not only identify the present risk but also consider the impact of these dynamic factors on the service user's level of risk at any point in time. These dynamic risk factors can also be protective especially in the case where a service user has all of the following:

- the skills and psychological resources to cope;
- meaningful work;
- a social network that is supportive;
- access to the required services.

Communication

Background

A mental health nurse is expected to demonstrate compassion when delivering care as well as being an effective communicator. Unlike most healthcare relationships the therapeutic relationship in mental health care is both the medium for treatment and, in most cases, the main treatment. Being an effective communicator gives the mental health nurse a platform from which to deliver a range of psychological interventions tailored to meet the specific needs of the mental health service user. Good communication is also pivotal in the establishment and continuation of a therapeutic relationship that manages risk, is recovery focused and has positive outcomes.

It is important to recognise that the more effective a mental health nurse's communication skills the more effective the nurse will be in delivering care. Communication should be seen as a two-way process in which information is shared between the service user and the mental health nurse; other people (including carers, relatives who are not carers, health professionals, health and social care professionals, social care staff, volunteers and befrienders) or agencies may also be part of this process. At times sharing information can be disrupted or blocked by a number of factors. In these situations the responsibility lies with the mental health nurse as the practitioner to firstly understand why this has happened and to secondly develop strategies to overcome any identified communication difficulties.

Professional skills

Mental health nurses should:

- have excellent communication, interpersonal and therapeutic skills;
- be skilled in working in partnership with service users and carers;
- engage in person-centred care that is compassionate and empowering;
- preserve dignity, be anti-discriminatory and practise within the law, considering such issues as confidentiality and consent.

Types of communication

Communication can be broken down into verbal communication and non-verbal communication. Verbal communication contains three key elements:

- the spoken word — vocals;
- the way the spoken word is expressed — paralanguage;
- the way spoken word is perceived by the other person — meta-communication.

The majority of our communication, however, is conveyed through non-verbal communication or body language, such as:

- facial expressions;
- eye contact;
- gestures;
- posture;
- head movements;
- personal space;
- touch;
- appearance.

During the communication process the mental health nurse needs to be aware of their own body language and its impact upon the service user. Nurses also have to be able to understand the potential messages that the other person's body language is conveying: is the service user angry; are they sad; do they look confused? The mental health nurse will, at times, need to adapt their body language; for example, if a service user is angry the mental health nurse will adopt a non-threatening but assertive posture.

Listening and responding

An important part of the communication process is actively listening to what the service user is saying and then responding appropriately. As an active listener the mental health nurse must concentrate on what the service user is saying; they must also control any potential distractions, giving the service user time and space to talk. The mental health nurse demonstrates that they are listening by responding in way that is appropriate to what is being said. This can be achieved through the mental health nurse nodding their head, a non-verbal sign that they are listening, summarising what the service user has said, and then checking and clarifying with the service user that their understanding of what has been said is correct. A key part of understanding requires the mental health nurse to be skilled in asking open questions (e.g. tell me about feeling sad) and also to be able to ask probing questions (e.g. what time of day do you feel most sad?).

The 6Cs

People with mental health needs can be at their most vulnerable, so it is essential in this situation that the mental health nurse shows empathy through a genuine understanding of the service user's experiences. In other words, they needs to engage in and promote person-centred care which is first and foremost compassionate in nature. By being an effective and compassionate communicator the mental health nurse will have a good foundation of skills, values and behaviours from which they can develop and deliver a range of psychological interventions. These baseline communication skills, values and behaviours are known as the 6Cs (CBCNO and DoH CAN 2012):

- care — service users receiving care expect it to be appropriate for them, whatever the circumstances;
- compassion (sometimes described as intelligent kindness) — how service users perceive the delivery of the care they receive;
- competence — the expertise, clinical and technical knowledge to deliver effective care at the right time;
- communication — an effective and central part of a successful therapeutic relationship, inclusive of all partners in the care-delivery process;
- courage —doing the right thing at the right time for the service users, including speaking up when they have concerns;
- commitment — placing service users and carers at the centre of a therapeutic relationship, driven by the service users' needs.

Diagnosis and classification

Background

Psychiatrists predominately classify mental distress as mental illness when the distress is greater than the statistical norm. Mental illness is further categorised into statistically agreed groupings or classifications, including:

- addictive disorders;
- anxiety disorders;
- eating disorders;
- mood disorders;
- neurocognitive disorders;
- neurodevelopmental disorders;
- personality disorders;
- psychotic disorders;
- sexual disorders;
- sleep disorders.

These disorders are further defined through a diagnostic process which is supported by internationally agreed frameworks and classification systems. It is important to acknowledge that psychiatric diagnoses do not fit as easily into the practice of the mental health nurse as into the practice of the psychiatrist. For mental health nurses a fundamental problem with applying diagnostic classifications is that classifying or applying labels is not holistic enough to identify all the needs of a mental health service user. However, mental health nurses have to be able to understand and work with this system because diagnosis and classification is a fundamental form of communication throughout mental health care.

Professional skills

Mental health nurses should:

- recognise different forms of mental distress and respond effectively irrespective of age or setting;
- understand the impact that different forms of mental distress can have upon an individual's ability to function;
- apply and value the use of evidence about appropriate interventions for different forms of mental distress and mental disorders;
- have an in-depth understanding of how different mental disorders need to be considered during the care and treatment of individuals with mental health needs.

Classification

Classifying mental illnesses provides a scientific basis upon which the practice of psychiatry can be built. Classification also provides a framework that improves:

- the diagnostic process — both reliability and validity;
- communication — by providing a common language;

- treatment outcomes and clinical management — using common approaches.

There are two established frameworks for classifying mental disorders:

- International Classification of Diseases (ICD; WHO 2010);
- Diagnostic and Statistical Manual of Mental Disorders (DSM; APA 2013).

The ICD was established in 1993 and it is now in its 10th version, at the time of writing it is currently being revised with the 11th version planned for released in 2018. DSM was established in 1952, the 5th version was released in 2013 and is currently in the process of being implemented. Both frameworks are distinct but generally they complement each other. North America tends to use DSM and the rest of the world tends to use ICD. ICD is a requirement of the World Health Organization. DSM maps to ICD. Some psychiatrists in the UK prefer DSM and will diagnose using that classification system; at coding this is then converted to ICD.

Diagnosis

The diagnostic process comprises an assessment of the service user. This process has two distinct steps:

- the psychiatric history and mental state examination;
- the formulation of a treatment plan.

The first step provides the psychiatrist with baseline assessment information related to the service user, including the history of the presenting problem and mental experiences, together with a description of the service user's behaviour at the time the assessment took place. The second step, the formulation of a treatment plan, summarises what the issues are, and at this stage a diagnosis is usually applied by the psychiatrist using the ICD classification system or, on occasion, the DSM classification system. The treatment plan is then formulated based upon the best available evidence.

The role of the mental health nurse

Mental health nurses usually have the most direct contact with mental health service users. This unique position shapes the care that the mental health nurse delivers. The knowledge generated from being in this unique position should be used to complement the information gathered during the diagnostic process. Using a psychiatric diagnosis in isolation provides only limited information, as it does not inform the mental health nurse how to support the service user at a person-centred level. On this basis the nurse needs to pay attention to the service-user's narrative and deliver any subsequent interventions through a collaborative and therapeutic relationship. These interventions should be:

- underpinned by psychological methods and theory;
- clinically effective and, where possible, evidenced based;
- person centred;
- focused on considering values and meanings.

Documentation

Background

Keeping a record of the planning and delivery of care is an important and essential part of mental health nursing practice. Records should provide a clear and accurate description of the care-delivery process; in the UK they should also adhere to the Nursing & Midwifery Council's (NMC's) guidance on record-keeping. When recording care the mental health nurse will need to find a balance between their professional view of a given situation and the service user's view; the nurse will then need to find an agreed viewpoint. Employing a person-centred and collaborative approach will assist in this process.

Record-keeping is 'essential to the provision of safe and effective care' (NMC 2009). Records are also part of the communication process, and better communication generally means that a better quality of care delivered. For example, if a service user's condition is clearly and accurately recorded then other members of the care team should be able to detect whether there have been any changes to the service user's condition over time and then act accordingly. This is particularly important when there are constant changes to the personnel delivering care, such as in the case of shift-pattern working. As mental health nurses work in different settings, for example in inpatient and community settings, records are often kept in several different formats, including paper and electronic records. Whatever the format of the records, the principles of good record-keeping remain the same. Types of records include:

- handwritten clinical notes;
- emails and text messages;
- clinical letters;
- X-rays, laboratory reports and printouts;
- incident reports and statements;
- photographs and videos.

Professional skills

Mental health nurses should:

- ensure that they maintain records that are based on the best available evidence and that these records are accurate, clear and complete, whatever the format;
- participate fully in the care-planning process, including the completion of relevant documentation;

- document care that fully meets the service user's needs, including taking appropriate action where required;
- manage record-keeping in a way that adheres to the relevant professional and legal frameworks.

The function of documentation

Documentation is used in many contexts and for a number of purposes, such as:

- improving accountability;
- presenting and supporting the clinical decision-making process;
- supporting effective communication;
- providing documentary evidence of the care delivered;
- supporting the clinical risk-management process;
- supporting clinical audit and research, and the complaints process.

Documentation standards

In the UK a mental health nurse's clinical record-keeping should adhere to the NMC's guidance and standards. The following list is a summary of these standards; it is recommended that the guidance is read in full (NMC 2009):

- handwriting should be legible and all entries should be fully signed with the date and time;
- the entry should be accurate, factual and the meaning clear with no unnecessary jargon;
- professional judgment should be used to decide what should be recorded;
- information related to a service user's care should be fully recorded;
- records should not be altered and/or destroyed without the relevant authorisation;
- any authorised alteration must be fully signed with the original entry record still clearly readable or auditable;
- ensure that the record-keeping process adheres to the relevant professional and legal frameworks as well as national and local policies;
- service users and carers should, where appropriate, be involved in the record-keeping process;
- information that is not clinically relevant should not be kept;
- service users should be made aware that their clinical records may be seen by other people or agencies involved in their care.

Further to the NMC's documentation standards as outlined above, the NMC included the professional expectation that nurses should 'keep clear and accurate records relevant to their practice' (NMC 2015).

This expectation covers all records not just service-user records. To achieve this expectation the nurse should:

- complete all records at the time or as soon as possible after an event;
- identify any risks or problems that have arisen and record the steps taken to deal with them;
- complete all records accurately and without any falsification;
- attribute any entries to yourself; they need to be clearly written, dated and timed;
- take all necessary steps to ensure that all records are kept securely;
- collect, treat and store all data and research findings appropriately.

Improving record-keeping

It is essential that mental health nurses adhere to the professional guidance on record-keeping but they also need to reflect on how they can continually improve their practice. When engaging in this process of reflection it might be useful to consider:

- Does your entry provide accurate evidence of the standard of care delivered?
- Is your entry person centred?

Early intervention services

Background

Early intervention services are a specialist mental health service offering treatment and support for young people experiencing psychoses for the first time and during the first three years following diagnosis. Early intervention services are set up differently across the country but broadly they offer a service that consists of family therapy, individual cognitive behavioural therapy (CBT), art therapies and occupational activities to young people between the ages of 14 and 35 years.

The Early Intervention Service was set up as a result of an ever increasing evidence base that there is a poorer prognosis for psychosis and schizophrenia when onset is in childhood or adolescence (NICE 2009, 2014), and furthermore there is a strong argument that an early intervention promotes a better health outcome for young people. The strength of the Early Intervention Service is that it is designed to deliver support and evidence-based interventions in a 'normalising' environment as opposed to admitting a young person to a mental health inpatient ward.

There is a natural partnership between Child and Adolescent Mental Health Services, including early intervention services, and adult mental health providers; thus it is vital that any transition from one care provider to another is managed properly and in a supportive way.

Professional skills

Mental health nurses should:

- be able to work with service users of all ages working in a way that promotes positive and is inclusive;
- recognise and respond to the needs of all service users who come into their care, drawing on a range of recovery-focused psychosocial interventions;
- use effective relationship-building and communication skills to engage with and support service users distressed by hearing voices, experiencing distressing thoughts or experiencing other perceptual problems;
- assess and meet the full range of essential physical and mental health needs of service users of all ages who come into their care;
- help service users experiencing mental health problems to make informed choices about pharmacological and physical treatments.

Prevention

When a person presents within primary-care services as:

- distressed and with a decline in social functioning;
- with transient psychotic symptoms or symptoms that are suggestive of a possible psychosis;
- or with a first-degree relative with psychosis;

they should be referred immediately to specialist mental health services. Current clinical guidelines advise that when a person is considered to be at risk of developing a psychosis they should be offered:

- individual CBT with or without family intervention;
- other interventions in accordance with agreed clinical guidelines.

First episode

Current clinical guidelines advise that when a person is experiencing a first episode of psychosis early intervention services should offer:

- care irrespective of age or duration of the untreated psychosis;
- an assessment for post-traumatic stress disorder and other trauma reactions;
- a choice of antipsychotic medication.

Medication

Young people are often treated with antipsychotic medication and, as such, mental health nurses are required to monitor symptoms, side effects and adherence. Before starting an antipsychotic medication it is recommended that a series of physical health baseline assessments are completed. Mental health nurses should be competent in the basic physical health checks below:

- weight and height;
- waist and hip circumference;
- pulse and blood pressure;
- fasting blood glucose, HbA1c, blood lipid profiles and prolactin levels;
- assessment of movement disorders;
- assessment of nutritional status, diet and level of physical activity.

It is important to monitor and record any behavioural changes during the titration of an antipsychotic medication. Side effects must be monitored, particularly the emergence of movement disorders.

Psychoeducation
It is essential that mental health nurses work in a multidisciplinary way that is quite distinct from other mental health services. Working with families and/or educators is key to a successful episode of care for a young person, and psychoeducation is therefore a significant part of the mental health nurses' role. Psychoeducation focuses on providing an individual diagnosed with a psychosis with the necessary information and skills to manage the symptoms of their condition. Good communication and negotiating skills are key to facilitating this process.

Capacity
All mental health nurses working with young people should be able to assess capacity including 'Gillick Competence' as well as a knowledge of other legislation such as the *Mental Capacity Act*, *Mental Health Act 1983 (amended 2007)*, and *The Children Act 1989 (amended 2004)*.

Psychological interventions
Knowledge of the evidence base and current National Institute for Health and Care Excellence (NICE) guidelines in the UK are crucial to ensuring that young people are receiving the best possible interventions and care. Depending on expertise, CBT may well be a key competency of the mental health nurse. In almost all cases, knowledge of family therapy, counselling and other specific psychosocial interventions will be a fundamental aspect of the mental health nurse role. Attention to culture, ethnicity and social inclusion are paramount when working with all people; remember that stigma and discrimination can often occur amongst young persons in mental health services. Central to the success of all the skills mentioned above is the compassion and interpersonal skills of the mental health nurse, which will ultimately facilitate a therapeutic relationship.

Electroconvulsive therapy

Background

Electroconvulsive therapy (ECT) is a treatment for number of mental health conditions, and involves passing electrical currents through the brain with the intention of causing a seizure. Inducing convulsions to treat mental health conditions has been used for centuries; in recent times insulin was used and then electric shocks. During the 1950s short-acting anaesthesia and muscle relaxants were used during ECT which reduced muscle pain and fractures.

ECT was previously used for quite a few mental health conditions, but is now is indicated in the case of:

- severe depression;
- a severe and prolonged episode of mania that has not responded to treatment;
- moderate depression that has not responded to multiple drug treatments.

Cognitive impairment can be a side effect of treatment. Dependent on the balance of risk, and bearing in mind that ECT can be a lifesaving treatment, ECT is contraindicated in:

- raised intracranial pressure;
- cardiovascular disease;
- dementias;
- epilepsy;
- cervical spine disease.

Professional skills

Mental health nurses should:

- ensure that they have an in-depth knowledge of common mental health treatments;
- offer holistic care and, working as part of the multidisciplinary team, offer a range of treatment options of which ECT may form a part;
- assist individuals with mental health problems to make informed choices about treatments;
- provide education, information and support related to the provision of pharmacological and physical treatments.

Procedure

Prior to an ECT procedure the service user will have a full physical examination, their consent will be obtained; this process may need to be managed in the UK through the provisions in the *Mental Health Act 1983 (amended 2007)*, and the service user will then be nil by mouth from midnight of the day before the procedure (NICE 2003). During the procedure the service user will be given a short-acting general anaesthetic and then a muscle relaxant is administered and a tongue guard is place in the mouth. Two electrodes are placed on the service user's temples; usually on either side (bilateral) or occasionally one side (unilateral). A brief electrical pulse is delivered at a voltage that is above the service user's seizure threshold (whereupon a seizure is normally induced). Bilateral ECT is more effective than unilateral ECT; however unilateral ECT has fewer side effects.

Treatment course
Service users can be given 6 to 12 ECT treatments over 3 to 6 weeks. The course of treatment will normally be stopped if there is no improvement in the service user's symptoms after 6 to 8 treatments.

Side effects
Common side effects include:

* feeling tired and drowsy;
* headache;
* muscle ache;
* nausea;
* confusion;
* temporary memory impairment.

It is important to note that the service user may experience side effects from the anaesthetic, which include cardiovascular problems.

Consent
ECT is normally given if consent is obtained, irrespective of whether the service user is detained under the *Mental Health Act 1983 (amended 2007)*. If a service user refuses to consent, or is so unwell that they either cannot consent or do not have the capacity to consent, and the procedure is essential then ECT may still be given under certain conditions. Under the *Mental Health Act 1983 (amended 2007)* a second opinion is sought from an independent psychiatrist who will consult with the multidisciplinary team, the service users and their relative/s; the second opinion doctor will then make a decision on whether the service user should receive ECT.

Elimination

Background
Supporting mental health service users to meet to their own physical needs can be a sensitive issue, especially when dealing with bowel and bladder care. The majority of mental health service users will be able to meet their own 'elimination' needs independently, in which case the role of the mental health nurse will focus on providing support and advice when personal hygiene issues arise. When a service user is unable to meet their own elimination needs independently, however, the mental health nurse should offer effective care that respects and maintains dignity.

Assisting service users to manage their elimination needs requires not only a sensitive approach but it also requires the mental health nurse to work in partnership with the service user. For this assistance to be effective the mental health nurse has to obtain consent, and when a service user is unable to provide consent their rights need to be protected. The type of assistance provided might range from prompting and reminding an individual to go to the toilet, to providing equipment such as commodes or bedpans. If physical assistance is required, whether this is with or without equipment, a manual handling assessment needs to be undertaken. It also has to be recognised that, although most individuals have a bowel and bladder routine, this routine can be quite specific to the individual and their circumstances.

Professional skills
Mental health nurses should:

- provide safe, person-centred care for service users who are unable to meet their own physical needs;
- act with dignity and respect to ensure that service users who are unable to meet their own physical needs feel empowered;
- deliver care that meets service user's essential needs, such as bowel and bladder care;
- work collaboratively to ensure an adequate fluid intake and output.

Elimination assessment
Elimination is the excretion of urine and faecal matter from the body. When assessing service user's bowel and bladder routine it is important to note the level of support they require and whether they have any concerns. Other types of information you might collect are the:

- frequency, volume, consistency and colour;
- presence of blood, mucus, undigested food or offensive smell;
- report of pain and/or discomfort;
- sample for urinalysis.

Incontinence
Incontinence is an inability to control the function of the bladder or bowel, which can be due to a dysfunction and/or underlying health problem. In most cases incontinence can be managed effectively through a continence management and treatment regime. Types of incontinence include:

- stress incontinence — a leakage of urine that usually happens during physical activity;
- urge incontinence — an uncontrollable urge to pass urine and at times an individual may find it difficult to make it to the toilet in time;

- overflow incontinence — an individual uncontrollably passes small amounts of urine during the day and night;
- reflex incontinence — a complete leakage of urine without the individual having a feeling of needing to go to the toilet or having control;
- constipation — when the stools become difficult to pass;
- faecal incontinence — when there is a loss control of the bowels.

Assisting with elimination

When managing incontinence the nurse might need to consider if a service user's continence could be due to mobility difficulties or the fact that they do not understand their surroundings. Some ward environments manage these issues by having good signage and by undertaking ward rounds every two hours. During rounds the nurses routinely engage with the service users, focusing on personal care including bladder and bowel care. This does not mean that a service user's specific elimination needs are not dealt with outside of these times. While undertaking bowel and bladder care the nurse must remember to:

- wear disposable gloves;
- wash hands even if wearing gloves;
- wash the service user;
- keep the skin clean;
- use a barrier cream sparingly and preferably use a cream that has a pH near to that of normal skin (pH5.5);
- not use solutions that contain alcohol or disinfectant.

Within a home environment the mental health nurses should work with other agencies to ensure that a service user's independence is maintained. This might include adapting the environment so that a service user has easy and safe access to toileting facilities.

Infection control

Background

Mental health nurses deliver many different clinical interventions, the majority of which are psychosocial. Yet it is easy to forget that mental health nurses are at times required to provide physical health care, such as clinical observations and wound care amongst many other interventions. When delivering these interventions it is important that the mental health nurse follows principles that focus on preventing and controlling infections.

Infection-control measures aim to have a zero tolerance of infection; mental health nurses have a key role to play in achieving this aim. It is also important to remember that when delivering physical health care there is always a risk, including that of cross-infection; the mental health nurse will need to manage these risks. One aspect of managing this risk is to implement effective infection-control procedures; the other aspect requires the mental health nurse to frame their practice through the risk-management process.

Professional skills
Mental health nurses should:

- adhere to local and national policies on the prevention and control of infection;
- apply agreed infection-control and prevention practices in all environments;
- provide effective nursing care in the case of infectious diseases, including the use of isolation techniques;
- act to reduce risk when handling sharps, contaminated linen and clothing, and when dealing with spillages of body fluid.

Physical health interventions
Mental health nurses deliver a number of physical health interventions that require the nurse to think about infection control and prevention. The following is an illustrative list of some of those interventions:

- taking a pulse;
- measuring blood pressure;
- taking a temperature;
- administering wound care;
- administering injections;
- collecting a sputum sample;
- measuring a peak flow rate;
- collecting urine for urinalysis;
- testing for blood glucose levels;
- administering first aid;
- administering basic life support.

Spreading of infections
Microorganisms can be spread in different ways, including by:

- aerosol;
- droplet;
- faecal–oral means;
- person-to-person contact, most often by contaminated hands;
- indirect contact, such as through food, water and inanimate objects;
- body fluids;
- insects and parasites.

Infection-control practices

There is a currently a national initiative to ensure that infection-control practices are consistent whatever the environment (RCN 2012). This is important for mental health nurses as they can practice within a wide variety of health and social care settings. The emphasis of the initiative is to maintain standards through training and to establish systems that ensure consistent and reliable practice, and there is a focus on clinical leaders acting as infection-control role models. To maintain consistency with this initiative mental health nurses need to:

- receive training on the standard principles of effective infection control and prevention;
- adhere to local and national reporting procedures for infections;
- manage and monitor the prevention and control of infection using a robust-risk-assessment process;
- provide and maintain a clean and a safe care environment;
- provide user-friendly and accurate information on infections and infection control to service users and carers;
- ensure that service users who have developed an infection receive care that aims to reduce the risk of passing the infection on to others;
- access laboratory support as appropriate.

Infection-control skills

Effective infection prevention and control ensures that the people who access health and social care services receive safe care. On this basis mental health nurses should be trained in:

- hand hygiene;
- personal protective equipment;
- safe use and disposal of sharps;
- aseptic technique.

Leadership

Background

It is easy to think that leadership is defined by being in a specific leadership role when, in reality, it is can be defined by assuming an informal leadership role when care delivery dictates. For example, a nurse might take a lead role within a multidisciplinary team meeting when advocating a specific treatment on behalf of a service user. At a professional level, leadership is a developmental journey whereby the nurse is able to contribute positively to the delivery of high-quality care.

Effective leadership within health and social care is a key component in the drive to improve care quality. To do this mental health nurses must be able to work in partnership with individuals living with mental health problems, and also with other professionals and external agencies. During this process to improve care quality they must also be able to utilise leadership skills, behaviours and values which include:

- being able to communicate effectively;
- dealing constructively with setbacks;
- taking on board others' viewpoints;
- being clear about the way forward;
- engendering trust.

Depending on the situation, the mental health nurse might use different leadership styles. For example, in an emergency situation an autocratic or directive style might be more appropriate than first seeking everyone's view (democratic style) or just allowing everyone to do their own thing (a laissez-faire style).

Professional skills
Mental health nurses should:

- be able to manage themselves and others to ensure that the quality of care and the safety of the service user are maintained or enhanced;
- be self-aware and professionally accountable, using clinical governance processes to maintain and improve practice standards;
- work effectively across professional and agency boundaries to create and maximise opportunities to help improve care delivery;
- actively participate in further developing their management and leadership skills through structured reflection.

Models of leadership
There are a number of theories and models of leadership, including:

- traits-based leadership — leaders are born not made, and they are born with the personality traits to be leaders;
- leadership as a behavioural style — leadership behaviours should be applied dependent on the situation; for example, some situations might require the leader to demonstrate decisiveness other situations might not;
- situational-contingency approaches to leadership — a leader is required to adapt their leadership style to suit the situation or circumstances; at times they might be required to be an authoritarian team leader and at other times they might seek the advice of the team;
- transformational approaches — a leader focuses on enhancing the performance of the individuals they lead through a number of different approaches, such as motivating individuals, providing a vision or direction, and through being a role model.

Improving practice

Clinical leadership should focus on continually improving the quality care delivered to mental health service users, irrespective of whether a mental health nurse's leadership role is an informal or formal role. To establish a strong foundation for being an effective clinical leader it is useful if the mental health nurse develops their practice to a level where they can cope skilfully with a range of clinical situations. Building on this foundation through lifelong learning the mental health nurse as a leader should consider cultivating the following qualities:

- effective self-management;
- integrity;
- having a focus on quality;
- motivation;
- influencing others;
- being adaptable and astute;
- being an agent for change;
- being authentic;
- being a coach.

The roles of mental health nurse and clinical leader use similar skills, values and qualities. To ensure that these are cultivated and directed in the right direction the mental health nurse, both as a practitioner and as a leader, should actively engage in:

- lifelong learning;
- expert skill development;
- critical reflection.

Emotional intelligence

Emotional intelligence is an important leadership skill. By being emotionally intelligent the mental health nurse has the ability to be emotionally aware of their feelings and the feelings of others. In addition, they can work with this emotional information to guide themselves and others appropriately. Emotional intelligent leaders have five characteristics:

- they are self-aware;
- they can control their emotions appropriately;
- they are motived and highly productive;
- they are empathetic;
- they have strong social skills.

Lifelong learning

Background

Mental health nurses should be committed lifelong learners who utilise the reflective process to explore, appreciate and develop their practice experiences. Continuing professional development (CPD) is a key part of the nurse's lifelong learning journey; however, lifelong learning is a wider concept that also takes into account personal learning which or may not relate to a nurse's professional practice. CPD, when actively underpinned by effective reflective practices, will help the nurse become an expert in their practice and has the benefit of improving the care that they deliver. It is important to recognise that because each nurse's experiences are unique then their lifelong learning journey will be unique and also dynamic. Being unique does not mean that formal education has no part to play in this journey, it just means that formal and informal learning should be utilised so that they complement each other.

In terms of mental health nursing the concept of lifelong learning is used to describe the expectation that mental health nurses will keep their skills and knowledge up-to-date throughout their working life. More formally, and at a professional level, lifelong learning is entwined with the process of CPD. On this basis, the Nursing & Midwifery Council in the UK has set a number post-registration education and practice (Prep) standards for CPD. These standards assist the mental health nurse to:

- provide a high standard of care;
- keep up-to-date with new practice developments;
- think and reflect;
- demonstrate that they are up-to-date and are developing their practice.

Professional skills
Mental health nurses should:

- keep their knowledge and skills up-to-date by learning from experience, through supervision, feedback, reflection and evaluation in a process of CPD;
- demonstrate a commitment to their own and others' lifelong learning and professional development;
- facilitate others, including nursing students, to develop their competence, using a range of professional and personal development skills;
- as both team member and team leader, actively seek and learn from feedback to enhance care delivery.

Post-registration education and practice standards
The Prep standards are legal requirements set by the NMC, and to which the nurse must adhere in order to maintain and renew their registration. Two standards are articulated in *The Prep handbook* (NMC 2011) as follows:

- the practice standard requires the nurse to have practised in some capacity by virtue of their nursing qualification for a minimum of 450 hours during the three years prior to the renewal of their registration. If the nurse does not meet this requirement they will need to undertake an approved return to practice course before they can renew their registration.
- the CPD standard includes a commitment to undertake at least 35 hours of learning activity relevant to their practice during the three years prior to their renewal of registration; to maintain a personal professional profile of their learning activity; and to comply with any request from the NMC to audit how they have met these requirements.

The Prep standards will be superseded by the revalidation standards when they come into effect in April 2016. Revalidation as a process is currently being piloted and the evaluation of these pilots will inform the implementation of these standards. For more information on the NMC's revalidation process, please see http://www.nmc.org.uk/standards/revalidation/

Expert practice

By maintaining and continually improving their practice the mental health nurse is engendering an opportunity to develop their expertise. The benefit of becoming an expert mental health nurse is that they are more effective than novice nurses when managing clinical situations that are ambiguous, complex and have no certain outcome (Smith 2012, 2014). This does not mean that the novice nurse or newly qualified mental health nurse will not be able to cope with a range of situations; at first they will simply not be as practised in dealing with situations as the expert mental health nurse. The knowledge and wide range of skills of the expert nurse are built through a number of stages in their development; these stages are described in the seminal work of Benner (1982) and include:

1. Learning to be a registered nurse (novice).
2. Starting to use practical experiences to contextualise knowledge.
3. Managing standard clinical situations but lacking in speed and flexibility.
4. Recognising and understanding non-standard situations.
5. Managing situations using both scientific and naturalistic knowledge (expert).

Reflection is key to being an expert; the process of reflection enables the nurse to develop their self-awareness to a level where they are able to clearly identify both their strengths and the areas that they need to develop further. It is important to recognise that knowledge accrued through the reflective process is especially useful as it is based upon experience. Similar to scientific knowledge, experienced-based knowledge should not be used in isolation, but rather it should be used to complement scientific knowledge to link both forms of knowledge directly to the nurses ongoing practice experience.

Managing aggression and violence

Background

Managing violence and aggression refers to managing behaviours that can result in harm to another person. This behaviour can be verbal and/or non-verbal, injury may or may not be sustained, and the intention to injure may or may not be clear.

Mental health nurses manage violence and aggression as part of managing risk, and the overwhelming focus is on prevention rather just intervening when an incident occurs. Incidents of violence and aggression, including assaults, are more likely to happen within inpatient settings. The factors behind these incidents include:

- the individual service user is highly impulsive;
- poor staff attitudes and behaviours — especially poor communication skills;
- inaccessible staff;
- locked wards;
- lack of privacy for service users;
- overstimulation — busy environments;
- understimulation — lack of activity;
- inconsistency in setting limits for what is and is not acceptable.

Professional skills

Mental health nurses should:

- work with service users in a way that that values and respects the person irrespective of their behaviour;
- prioritise actions that enhance the service user's safety and psychological security by taking a positive risk-management approach that is seamless across all services;
- use effective communication skills when dealing with even the most challenging situations, including emergencies, unexpected occurrences, complaint, disputes, conveying unwelcome news, and de-escalating aggression;
- recognise the signs of aggression and react appropriately, keeping themselves and others safe;
- select and apply appropriate strategies and techniques for conflict resolution, de-escalation and physical intervention (restraint).

Reducing incidents

To reduce incidents of violence and aggression the mental health nurse will need to carry out a comprehensive risk assessment as required (e.g. on admission to services and on a regular basis while in services, and when there is a change in circumstances, such as becoming unwell or exhibiting risky behaviour). The risk assessment should identify following:

- history of aggression;
- trigger factors;
- history of abuse;
- previous risk-management plans.

When managing inpatient settings the staff teams should take a strengths approach to risk, recognising the need to work therapeutically in a positive and enabling manner.

The environment

Being a service user on an inpatient ward can be frustrating, especially when restrictions are applied to movement and/or behaviour. Although these restrictions are applied in the best interest of the service user they can still feel coerced and it is therefore important that the service user is supported to communicate their needs and feelings in a healthy way. Providing an environment that offers the appropriate psychological therapies and psychosocial interventions is important; however, just as important is the need to offer other structured activities such as:

- physical pursuits;
- leisure time and leisure activities;
- leave — both escorted and unescorted;
- occupational activities;
- quiet time and space.

The inpatient environment should also:

- be clean with bright and friendly decor;
- provide outside space that is easily accessible;
- provide private spaces, including storage for personal items;
- bedrooms that promote sleep and are easy to personalise.

In addition inpatient settings can, at times, be intimating and bullying, amongst other things, can take place. The staff team need to work together identify and managing these potential problems in a way that is supportive but also sets acceptable limits on behaviour, attitudes and values.

Training

To manage violence and aggression effectively mental health nurses working in all settings need to be supported to continually develop their emotional intelligence and leadership skills. Mental health nurses will also need to develop the following knowledge and skills:

- values-based practice;
- understand the risk factors that increase the incidences of violence and aggression;
- de-escalation:
  - recognising the signs of aggression;
  - using effective communication in all circumstances;
  - using distraction and relaxation techniques.
- break-away techniques;
- restraint — always used as a last resort;
- post-incident debriefing (a structured format);
- post-incident reviews (unstructured format);
- medication — the appropriate use of rapid tranquillisation medication when required.

Community

When working in the community for a community team it is important the mental health nurse follows the organisation policy on lone working in order to minimise their risk of experiencing aggression or violence.

Managing people

Background

Part of the role of the mental health nurse is to manage others; this may be in a formal or informal capacity. Before the nurse starts to manage others they first have to be able to manage themselves, and key to this is self-awareness. By being self-aware the nurse is not only aware of their own thoughts and feelings, but they should, in time, also be able to understand how these affect others. As the nurse becomes skilled in understanding themselves and others then the next stage is to use this knowledge to influence and facilitate positive change. During this process the nurse will also become assertive, whereby they are neither aggressive (i.e. impose their will on others) nor submissive (i.e. allow others to impose their will on them).

During recent times the formal role of managing nursing teams has become more complex. Not only are there many different nursing management roles but it is not always clear from a title what a nurse manager does or does not manage. Management roles within health and social care can also change almost overnight.

There are some common management functions, however, including the following:

- managing the performance of a team and the individuals within that team;
- delegation;
- resolving conflict;
- managing change;
- decision-making.

At an informal level, for example when a nurse is part of a team but is acting as a leader by advocating for a service user, the nurse needs to be an effective influencer. This is especially the case when they need to change the attitudes of others to gain an agreed position or way forward. Influencing skills include:

- active listening and questioning;
- persuasion;
- being assertive.

Professional skills
Mental health nurses should:

- manage themselves and others effectively;
- work collaboratively with mental health service users, carers, other professionals and agencies to enhance care delivery;
- engage actively in lifelong learning both as a practitioner and as a leader to enhance care;
- assertively challenge bad or sloppy practice in self and others,
  - act as an effective role model and as an effective clinical supervisor during the care-delivery process.

People-management skills
Managing people can be stressful but it can also be rewarding; the key to being effective in this role is preparation. This can take the form of a formal course and/or being mentored while developing effective people-management skills. The types of skills the mental nurse should develop include:

- being a role model;
- actively listening to people;
- communicating a clear vision of the way forward;
- being adaptive — using different skills for different situations;
- making assertive decisions;
- enabling people to make decisions;
- taking systematic approach to problem-solving;
- being emotionally intelligent.

Coaching and mentoring

During their day-to-day role mental health nurses will support and mentor students. Mentoring is a process whereby the nurse supports a student to achieve a number of set goals. To do this the nurse will facilitate the student's learning through a systematic process during which they will:

- role model a skill;
- give the student an opportunity to practice the skill safely;
- support the student to carry out the skill in live practice;
- provide structured feedback;
- engage the student in critical thinking.

Coaching is a similar process, although there is less focus on teaching and more focus on improving performance through an action-focused dialogue. The coaching relationship gives the coachee the opportunity to have protected space to focus on their development, which is similar in some aspects to the clinical supervision process/relationship. The mental health nurse as a coachee may utilise this approach to develop their own people-management skills or they may coach others. Coaching can also be used as way of ensuring that coachees are accountable for their development through the setting of agreed actions and outcomes; coaching can also be used to support individuals through change. A typical coaching session/process is outlined below:

1. establish trust between the coach and the coachee through an agreed contract;
2. agree a developmental plan and set achievable goals and timescales;
3. implement the development plan;
4. evaluate progress.

Managing change

Change can have an emotional impact that needs to be managed by a leader who is sensitive to this emotional context. One way to doing this is to seeing the role of managing people through change as more about managing relationships and building support than just driving through change. In this situation the mental health nurse needs to engage in a discussion with the individuals they manage in a way that promotes negotiation and agreement, but is also:

- collaborative;
- productive;
- positive.

Managing risk

Background

Mental health nurses are required to manage clinical risk, though there is a tendency to focus on a service user's risk to self and others rather than seeing risk as a wider issue. Clinical risk management in a wider context focuses on keeping service users safe; to do this you have to be able to identify potential hazards and risks. Within mental health care the nurse also has to take in consideration that managing clinical risk should be a process that is partnership focused.

Risk relates to the threat or likelihood that an adverse action or event will occur. Therefore, clinical risk management is concerned with the development of strategies that prevent such an action or event from occurring, or if prevention is not possible the focus is on minimising harm/s. Hazards and risks can include events that involve not only service users but also staff and carers. These events include deliberate self-harm and violence to others, slips and falls, and also administrative errors that may have a negative impact upon care.

Professional skills

Mental health nurses should:

- recognise risk;
- manage risk in a way that is person centred and recovery focused;
- be aware of the potential risks of the care they deliver;
- report concerns promptly and change care when required to maintain safety;
- manage risk both independently and as part of a team approach.

Risk

Risks are adverse incidents that are waiting to happen, whereas a hazard is something that has the potential to cause harm, such as a spillage on a floor that has not been dealt with. Clinical risk refers to risk within a care-delivery context. Use of the term risk with a narrow definition tends to focus on the potential for clinical errors rather than enabling the nurse to manage risk holistically. It is therefore important that risk is framed in terms of a managed and holistic process. Mental health nurses tend to use the language of risk in a holistic way that includes hazards; risk is also used to refer to the potential of something going wrong when delivering care. Risks can include:

- medication incidents;
- consent and capacity incidents;
- control and restraint incidents;

- breaches in confidentiality;
- accidents to staff, service users and visitors;
- environmental incidents such as flood and fire.

Risk management

Risk management is a systematic process of identifying and then managing risk through preventing, eliminating or minimising the identified risk. The steps of a risk-management process are to:

1. identify the risk and its relationship to care outcomes;
2. analyse the potential impact of the risk;
3. evaluate the risk, considering benefits and potential costs;
4. review: what has been learnt in the process of managing risk?

In terms of nursing practice the mental health nurse needs to have systems in place that focus on keeping themselves and the people they work with safe. The risk-management process also requires the mental health nurse to learn from their experiences of adverse incidents and change their behaviour to reduce the potential of the event occurring again. Learning from incidents both at an individual level and at an organisational level requires the mental health nurse to be effective in how they communicate and also document the issues that have arisen.

Risk and organisational culture

Risk management is not just about preventing risk; for an organisation to grow it must, at times, take risks but these risks need to be identified and managed. For example, on the basis of evidence that seems to show a benefit, an NHS Trust might want to introduce a new psychological intervention into the care of people living with dementia. Before introducing this intervention the Trust needs to identify the risks and the benefits; if they decide to go ahead they need to develop an action plan that manages those identified risks.

Clinical governance

Risk management is a component of clinical governance, which is a process or system whereby healthcare organisations are required to keep improving the quality of the services they provide. To do this organisations are required to safeguard high standards of care through promoting a working environment in which excellent care will grow. For clinical governance to work effectively there must be:

- clinical governance policies and procedures in place, which also include the management of risk;
- clear lines of responsibility and accountability;
- quality improvement systems in place;
- education and training plans;
- procedures to identify and manage concerns about the quality of care.

In addition to risk management, clinical governance as a process will usually include the following elements:

- education and training — ensuring staff have up-to-date skills and knowledge;
- clinical audit — measuring the performance of clinical practice against agreed standards;
- research and development — creating a culture of practice that is underpinned by robust evidence;
- candour — supporting staff to be open and willing to discuss poor practice and near misses;
- information management — collecting good quality information.

Medication

Background
When working with a mental health service user mental health nurses will deliver a number of nursing interventions; it is not unusual for the administration of psychiatric medication to be one of these interventions. On this basis it is important for the mental health nurse to not only understand what they are administrating but also to know how medication fits with the other interventions that they provide. The nurse also needs to be an educator, which means being able to provide information to individuals with mental health problems about the medication they have been prescribed.

Psychiatric medication is licensed medication that exerts a desired effect on the brain and nervous system. These medications can be prescribed for a range of mental disorders; they usually form part of a package of care that also includes psychological approaches.

Professional skills
Mental health nurses should:

- ensure that they have an in-depth knowledge of common mental health treatments including medication;
- offer holistic care and, working as part of the multidisciplinary team, offer a range of treatment options of which medicines may form a part;
- assist individuals with mental health problems to make informed choices about the pharmacological treatments they might receive;
- provide education, information and support related to the provision of pharmacological treatments.

Types of psychiatric medication
The main groups of psychiatric medication are:

- antidepressant drugs;
- antipsychotic drugs;

- anxiolytic and hypnotic drugs;
- mood stabilisers;
- anti-dementia drugs.

Antidepressant drugs

Antidepressant drugs are used to treat depression, usually moderate to severe depression. It is thought that they work by increasing the transmission of the monoamines (serotonin, noradrenaline and occasionally dopamine) in the brain. There are a number of categories of antidepressants and different categories cause different side effects. Common side effects include:

- nausea and dizziness;
- sexual dysfunction;
- drowsiness;
- insomnia;
- dry mouth;
- constipation;
- agitation and irritability.

Antipsychotic drugs

Antipsychotic drugs are used to treat the symptoms of psychosis, such as delusions, hallucinations and thought disorder. It is thought that they reduce the symptoms of psychosis by blocking the dopamine (D2/3) receptors in the brain. There are two categories of antipsychotic drugs: the typical antipsychotic drugs and the atypical antipsychotic drugs. Both categories of antipsychotic drugs have a number of side effects that include:

- movement disorders;
- sedation;
- weight gain.

The side effects of atypical antipsychotic drugs commonly include:

- weight gain;
- feeling sluggish;
- impaired glucose intolerance;
- hypersalivation, constipation, nausea (these side effects are generally only attributable to clozapine).

The side effects of typical antipsychotics commonly include:

- stiffness and shakiness (parkinsonism);
- feeling sluggish and slow;
- restlessness (akathisia);
- postural hypotension;
- sexual dysfunction;
- breast swelling or tenderness.

Anxiolytic and hypnotic drugs

Benzodiazepines are the most commonly used category of drugs in this group, and have both anxiolytic and hypnotic effects. They are effective for the short-term treatment of generalised anxiety, insomnia, alcohol withdrawal states and the control of violent behaviour. They work by increasing the inhibitory effects of γ-aminobutyric acid in the brain, and thereby induce sleep and muscle relaxation. Another anxiolytic drug buspirone is used in the short-term treatment of anxiety. Hypnotic drugs, such as zopiclone and zolpidem have a similar action to the anxiolytic drugs, but without the muscle relaxation. Common side effects of anxiolytic and hypnotic drugs include:

- dizziness;
- drowsiness;
- impaired coordination;
- memory impairment;
- dependence and withdrawal symptoms.

Mood stabilisers

Lithium is a mood stabiliser used in the treatment of recurrent bipolar affective disorder; its mechanism of action is unknown. Lithium can be toxic above a certain dose range; its optimal range is 0.4–1.0 mmol/L). Monitoring of the service user before commencement of the drug should include thyroid and renal function tests, repeated 6 months thereafter. In addition, lithium should be taken weekly initially and then every 12 weeks. Other mood stabilisers include sodium valproate and carbamazepine; although their precise modes of action are unknown, they tend to reduce excitability within the manic phase. Side effects of lithium include:

- nausea;
- fine tremor;
- weight gain;
- urinary problems;
- skin problems.

Signs of lithium toxicity include:

- vomiting;
- diarrhoea;
- coarse tremor;
- slurred speech;
- drowsiness;
- confusion.

Anti-dementia drugs

Donepezil, rivastigmine, galantamine and memantine are used in the early (mild to moderate) stages of dementia. Side effects include:

- diarrhoea;
- muscle cramps;

- fatigue;
- nausea and vomiting;
- weight loss;
- drowsiness.

Children

Psychiatric medication is frequently prescribed in the treatment of several psychiatric disorders in childhood, including nocturnal enuresis (bed wetting), attention deficit hyperactivity disorder, autism, sleep disorders, tic disorders, conduct disorders, anxiety disorders, depression and psychosis. It is important to recognise that children differ from adults in their ability to absorb, metabolise and eliminate drugs and should therefore be closely monitored while taking psychiatric medication.

Medicines management

Background

Medicines management is an important component of mental health nursing practice, especially when medication is utilised as the initial treatment. The term 'medicines management' encompasses not only the administration of medication, it also has a broader definition. As an example, medication can support the service user's journey to recovery but only if medicines management is viewed as a part of the therapeutic relationship. The value of this approach is that the service user is a collaborative partner in a process that aims to enable them to make autonomous decisions about their prescribed medication.

Administrating medication is an important part of medicines management. To ensure that mental health nurses safely and effectively administer medication they need to consider the issue of adherence. This issue is not unique to the mental health field; medication adherence is a major challenge for all healthcare professionals. If a person does not take their medication as prescribed it can impact adversely on their recovery as well as their health and well-being. Not adhering to a medication regime can be:

- unintentional — a person forgets to take their medication;
- intentional — a person decides not to take their medication.

To enhance adherence the mental health nurse should consider:

- providing education about medication and its role in treating and/or controlling the symptoms of the identified health condition;
- supporting the service user to shape their daily routine in a way that incorporates their medication regime; service users should also be encourage to talk about the drawbacks and the benefits of taking medication.

LIBRARY, UNIVERSITY OF CHESTER

Professional skills

Mental health nurses should:

- ensure that medicines management is built on safe and effective practice, supported by a commitment to work in partnership with the service user;
- administer medicines, and keep and maintain records that relate to medicines management in accordance with the relevant professional standards;
- ensure that their medicines management practice adheres to the relevant ethical–legal frameworks and also to the relevant national and local policy guidelines.

Medication management standards

When managing medicines mental health nurses in the UK should adhere to the Nursing & Midwifery Council's standards (NMC 2008). The following is a summarised list of those standards; it is recommended that the guidance is read in full:

- methods — medication must only be supplied and administered via a patient-specific direction or patient medicines administration chart;
- checking — any direction to administer a medicine must be checked;
- prescription medicines — only in exceptional circumstances and with certain conditions a nurse may label from stock and supply a clinically appropriate medicine;
- storage — all medicines should be stored in accordance with their UK license;
- transportation — nurses may transport medication to service users in certain cases and under certain conditions;
- administration — the nurse must be certain of the identity of the service user and that they are not allergic to the medicine; the nurse must know therapeutic uses of the medicine to be administered, its normal dosage, side effects, precautions and contraindications; the nurse must check the expiry date of the medicine and that the prescription is clearly written and unambiguous; the method of administration, route and timing must also be considered;
- assessment — the nurse is responsible for the initial and continued assessment of service users who are self-administering medication;
- remote prescription or direction to administer — in exceptional circumstances and under certain conditions the use of information technology (such as fax, text message or email) may be used;
- titration — when medication has been prescribed within a range of dosages, it is acceptable for nurses to titrate dosages;

- preparing medication in advance — a nurse must not prepare substances for injection in advance;
- nursing students — students must never administer or supply medicinal products without direct supervision;
- management of adverse effects — if a nurse makes an error they must take action to prevent any potential harm to the service user and report the incident as soon as possible.

Psychoeducation

Psychoeducation is a holistic approach that focuses on supporting the service user to develop healthy coping strategies. This approach involves collaborating with the service user to become more knowledgeable about their condition and treatment, including medication. By empowering the service user to become more knowledgeable the service user will better engage with their treatment and, in the long term, there will be more positive health-related outcomes. For example, when a service user with a severe and enduring mental health condition undergoes psychoeducation they start to adhere to their treatment, attend cognitive behavioural therapy sessions and take their medication as prescribed this, in turn, leads to the stabilisation of their mental health condition.

Mental health law

Background

On a day-to-day basis mental health nurses have to make practice decisions that are consistent with a number of legal frameworks. The added dimension in mental health nursing is that these decisions might include either restricting a mental health service user's freedoms or, where these restrictions are in place, maintaining the use of these restrictions. This does not mean that a mental health user does not have rights, however, it is quite the opposite, and it is therefore important that the mental health nurse knows how to balance autonomy of the service user against managing risk.

There are a number of legal frameworks that mental health nurses need to both work with and understand. Not all of these frameworks are specific to mental health care (for example, the *Human Rights Act 1998*) nonetheless, the mental health nurse must still be able to work with and understand these frameworks. The mental health nurse will work within a framework, such as the *Mental Health Act 1983 (amended 2007)* for England and Wales, that allows mental health nurses to restrict freedoms in certain circumstances. They will also work with legal frameworks that support individuals with severe mental problems to make decision, including the *Mental Capacity Act* 2005 which applies to England and Wales.

Professional skills

Mental health nurses should:

- understand and apply current legislation within their practice in way that protects vulnerable individuals;
- act within the law when collaboratively working with individuals living with mental health problems;
- respect and uphold a mental health service user's rights, acting in accordance with the law and relevant ethical and regulatory frameworks, including local protocols;
- know when to share personal information with others when the interests of safety and protection override the need for confidentiality.

The *Human Rights Act*

The *Human Rights Act 1998* came into full force in the UK in 2000. This Act protects the rights of the individual through a number of articles. All of the articles are relevant to individuals with mental health problems, but when an individual's freedoms are restricted the following articles have particular relevance:

- the right to life (article 2);
- the prohibition of torture (article 3);
- the right to liberty and security (article 5);
- the right to respect for private and family life (article 8).

The *Mental Capacity Act*

Individuals are generally presumed to have the capacity to make their own decisions, such as:

- understand information relevant to a decision;
- retain, use and weigh that information in the process of making that decision;
- communicate the decision.

When individuals lack capacity there is a supportive and transparent process enshrined within the *Mental Capacity Act*. This process acknowledges that a lack of capacity may be temporary and transient, and that individuals lacking capacity should, where possible, be helped to make their decisions. This Act applies to England and Wales; Scotland has similar legislation (the *Adults with Incapacity Act 2000*); Northern Ireland does not have specific legislation but relevant legislation includes the *Enduring Powers of Attorney Order 1987*.

The *Mental Health Act*

The *Mental Health Act 1983 (amended 2007)* of England and Wales is the legal framework under which an individual can be compulsory admitted, detained and treated in hospital. The Act includes provision for a community treatment order, whereby following discharge from a Section 3 or Section 37 admission an individual may be recalled back to hospital on certain grounds. The Act has civil and forensic sections.

Civil sections of the Mental Health Act 1983 (amended 2007)

The following is a brief overview of the main civil sections of the *Mental Health Act* 1983 *(amended 2007)* a mental health nurse will use; however there are other sections that the mental health nurse needs to be familiar with:

- Section 2 is an admission for assessment. Two doctors must make the recommendation and the application is then made by an approved mental health professional (AMHP). A Section 2 admission is for a maximum of 28 days.
- Section 3 is an admission for treatment. Two doctors must make the recommendation, and the application is then made by an AMHP. The duration of a Section 3 admission is six months; it can be renewed for a further six months, and thereafter for further periods of 12 months.
- Section 4 is an urgent assessment in the community. One doctor makes the recommendation. The duration of a Section 4 admission is 72 hours; with a second medical recommendation, however, a Section 4 admission can be converted to a Section 2 admission.
- Section 5 defines the holding powers of nurses and doctors when a service user is an inpatient. Section 5 (2) defines the doctors' holding power with a duration of 72 hours. Section 5 (4) defines the nurses' holding power and has a duration of 6 hours.
- Section 136 is implemented when a mentally disordered person is found in public place. A police constable can remove a mentally disordered person from a public place to a place of safety for 72 hours to enable a registered medical practitioner and an AMHP to assess the individual and, if required, make arrangements for admission.

Forensic sections of the Mental Health Act 1983
(amended 2007)

The following is a brief overview of the main forensic sections of the *Mental Health Act 1983 (amended 2007)* that a mental health nurse will use; however there are other sections that the mental health nurse needs to be familiar with:

- Section 35 is a remand for a report. This applies when the courts remand an accused individual to a hospital setting for a report on their mental condition.

- Section 36 is a remand for treatment. This applies when the courts remand an accused individual to a hospital setting for treatment of a mental condition.
- Section 37 is a hospital order. Similar to a Section 3, this applies when the courts impose a hospital order, usually after a conviction. When restrictions apply then a Section 41 is applied and this is known as a Section 37/41 — a hospital order with restrictions.
- Section 38 is an interim hospital order. This applies when the courts impose a hospital order for a convicted person to receive treatment for a mental condition before sentencing.
- Section 47 is a prison transfer to a hospital. This applies when a person is transferred to hospital for treatment of a mental condition. When restrictions apply this is known as a Section 47/49 — a transfer with restrictions.

Scotland

Scotland has similar legislation to the *Mental Health Act 1983 (amended 2007)* for England and Wales, known as the *Mental Health (Care and Treatment) (Scotland) Act 2003*. The main assessment and treatment orders are:

- emergency detention — urgent assessment for a duration of 72 hours;
- short-term detention — for detention in hospital for a duration of 28 days;
- compulsory treatment order — for detention in a hospital or the community for a duration of 6 months initially and renewable for a further 6 months, after which it can be renewed every 12 months;
- nurses' holding power, which has a duration of 2 hours;
- removal to place of safety by the police when an individual appears to be in mental distress and in a public place and is need of care and treatment;
- interim compulsion — a longer period of assessment made by the court with a duration of 1 year and renewable every 12 weeks;
- assessment — an assessment order for 28 days made by the court;
- treatment — a treatment order made by the court for the duration of the remand period or until sentencing.

Northern Ireland

In Northern Ireland the *Mental Health Order 1986* is still in effect; however, it will be replaced by the Mental Capacity Bill. The Order is divided into the following parts:

- Part 1 — definitions;
- Part 2 — the legal framework for compulsory admission;
- Part 3 — framework for persons with a mental disorder concerned in criminal proceedings;

- Part 4 — law on consent to treatment;
- Parts 5 and 6 — protections for persons with a mental disorder;
- Part 7 — registration of private hospitals;
- Part 8 — the management of property and affairs of patients;
- Part 9 — miscellaneous functions and statutory duties.

Monitoring

The use of these legal frameworks is monitored by Care Quality Commission in England, the Healthcare Inspectorate in Wales, the Mental Welfare Commission in Scotland, and the Regulation and Quality Improvement Authority in Northern Ireland.

Nutrition and fluid management

Background

Nutritional health is the foundation for good physical and mental well-being. It is generally recognised that mental health service users often have poor nutrition and a lack of physical activity. This may be caused by the social circumstances of the service user (for example, living in more deprived areas or finding it difficult to gain employment), but it may also be caused by the side effects of psychiatric medication. Whatever the causes are, it is known that mental health service users have an increased risk of mortality and physical illness (DoH 2011a). On this basis mental health nurses play a key role in promoting good nutritional health within their client group.

Maintaining a balanced diet, which includes drinking enough water, is essential for good health and well-being. When someone is physically unwell, depending on the condition and the circumstances, this can negatively impact upon their ability to maintain a balanced diet, and if the person then becomes malnourished this can adversely affect their recovery. Being malnourished can impair a person's immune response, it can delay wound healing and it can also increase the risk of mortality and developing other physical problems and illnesses (NICE 2006). To maintain a balanced diet a person needs the right amounts of the following:

- carbohydrates;
- proteins;
- fats;
- vitamins;
- minerals.

A specific issue within the field of mental health is weight gain. Service users treated with antipsychotic medication are more likely to be clinically obese than the general population (Nash 2014). This, in turn, can increase an individual's chances of developing diabetes and coronary heart disease. Taking this into consideration, when an individual commences antipsychotic treatment it is important that their weight is monitored regularly and action is taken where there are concerns about weight gain.

Professional skills
Mental health nurses should:

- assess and monitor diet and fluid status and, where required, formulate effective plans of care;
- support service users in choosing and maintaining a healthy nutritional diet and fluid intake;
- ensure that service users unable to take food and fluids by mouth receive adequate fluid and nutrition to meet their needs.

Assessing nutrition and fluid intake
Managing nutrition requires the mental health nurse to assess a service user's current nutritional status. This assessment should be part of a continuous process so that information can be compared over a period of time, which is particularly important when actual weight gain is identified over a specific time period. The type of information collected should include:

- body weight — then calculate the body mass index;
- waist-to-hip ratio;
- clinical examination/observations as appropriate — physical appearance, oedema, mobility, mood, wound healing;
- dietary intake over a 24 hour period;
- diet history such as food frequency, food habits, meal pattern, portion size and any eating difficulties.

Nutritional support
Within the inpatient setting nutritional support might range from providing a specific diet to assisting service users to eat and drink. The support provided will dependent on the service user's identified needs and their level of dependence. Interventions might include:

- diet modification, such as providing smaller and more regular meals, or increasing or reducing a specific food group;
- dietary supplements, such as specific vitamins and/or minerals;
- feeding a service user, where possible self-feeding should be encouraged and supported throughout;
- enteral tube feeding — providing a specific feed through a tube directly into the service user's gastrointestinal tract;
- intravenous fluids, which should be given when a service user is dehydrated.

When providing nutritional support it is important to recognise that a number of factors can impact upon a service user's ability to eat and drink independently. These can include:

- difficulty chewing and/or swallowing;
- weakness, stiffness or paralysis affecting the arms, hands and/or fingers;
- mobility problems that adversely affect a service user's ability to position themselves while eating.

Health promotion

When a service user is independent then nutritional support might take the form of promoting a good diet, which could include referring the service user to a dietician. It is important to note that changing a regular diet is a lifestyle change. With this in mind, the mental health nurse may be required to undertake motivational work to support the service user in their efforts to make a sustainable change to their eating habits. The health belief model (Nash 2014) is a model that has shaped the way nurses help people to change to a healthier lifestyle; at a practice level it has the following common features:

- recognising that there is a problem;
- understanding the risks of not changing;
- identifying the benefits of changing;
- recognising potential barriers to change.

Organising care

Background

Mental health nurses are professionally accountable for their own practice but they rarely work in isolation. Most mental health nurses will work as part of a multidisciplinary team, and they may also work as part of a nursing team. Within these different teams care-delivery decisions will be made and acted upon. During this process the mental health nurse needs to be both an effective team leader and an effective team member. They also need to ensure that the service user is at the centre of the decision-making process and ensure that the rights of the service user are fully respected.

Health and social care structures in the UK are constantly changing both at a national and at a local level. Organisational structures that are constantly changing can have an operational impact upon the way care is delivered. The role of the mental health nurse is to negotiate this constant change while delivering the best care available. An added challenge for the mental health nurse is the fluidity of organisational structures within the mental health field, especially when there is a greater focus on community working and multidisciplinary case management. The structure of an organisation is dependent on the aims of the organisation; for example, mental health NHS trusts aim to provide health and social care for individuals with mental health problems. This provision is delivered through a number of services that include:

- acute inpatient;
- assertive outreach;
- community mental health;
- crisis intervention;
- drugs and alcohol;
- early intervention;
- forensic;
- liaison psychiatry;
- outreach;
- rehabilitation.

Professional skills
Mental health nurses should:

- work as an autonomous and confident member of the multidisciplinary team, while promoting the continuity of care;
- safely lead, coordinate and manage care that is responsive to the needs of individuals living with mental health problems;
- deliver personalised care that is based on mutual understanding and respect for the individual's situation;
- maintain a safe environment and safeguard individuals living with mental health problems from vulnerable and potentially harmful situations.

Organising care delivery
Different models are used to organise mental health nursing care, but whichever model is used it should always aim to provide a good quality of care. Within an inpatient environment the delivery of this care is influenced by the multidisciplinary decision-making process; this may be via multidisciplinary team meetings or ward rounds. At an operational level nurses deliver the majority of this care and care delivery will be organised through a number of different approaches, although these approaches are not mutually exclusive:

- the task approach — the focus is on delivering a task, such as administrating medication or undertaking observations;
- the service-user allocation approach — a nurse is assigned to care for a specific number of service users;
- the team nursing approach — a team of qualified and unqualified nurses will care for a specific group of service users;
- the primary nursing approach — throughout their stay in hospital a service user will be cared for by a named qualified nurse who will be responsible and accountable for the coordination of their care.

A case management approach to care delivery is typically used within the community mental health team settings. This is a multidisciplinary team approach whereby the team is involved in both the decision-making process and the delivery of care, although in terms of overall responsibility one member of the team is allocated to be the case manager. Typically the case manager's role is to:

- undertake a comprehensive assessment;
- devise a person-centred care plan that manages risk;
- monitor progress and evaluate the plan of care accordingly;
- signpost to other services or members of the team when required;
- be an advocate for the service user.

Person-centred care

Whichever approach is used, nursing care delivery should be person centred, focusing on the service user's needs, strengths and preferences. Care delivery should also take into account that a service user may lack capacity and, in this case, the mental health nurse should follow the relevant legal framework and/or guidance.

Best practice

Mental health nurses working in partnership with service users who have complex needs are required to deliver high-quality care. During this process they also have to be able to influence external agencies successfully to ensure that a holistic and integrated package of care is implemented effectively. At the same time they have to make sense of a health and social care environment where structures are constantly changing. Using a model of care delivery will provide a sense of consistency when dealing with all of this change, although it is important that the nurse is skilful enough to be adaptive to different ways of working. On this basis the nurse will have to complement their baseline skills by engaging in a journey of lifelong learning where they clearly identify and then address their learning needs.

Physical well-being

Background

The role of the mental health nurse is to promote good physical health and well-being. This is especially important when considering that individuals diagnosed with a severe mental health problem are more likely to experience physical health problems than the general population (Nash 2014). The first stage of promoting good physical health and well-being is to ensure that an individual's physical health needs are identified. This process should take the form of regular physical assessments, and any needs identified should be addressed through an integrated and holistic package of care. Mental health nurses will also be required to deliver physical health care and/or signpost individuals to the appropriate services.

Physical health problems are common in individuals diagnosed with severe mental illness, such as depression, schizophrenia and bipolar affective disorder (Nash 2014). The most common types of physical health problems encountered by mental health nurses include:

- cardiovascular disease;
- respiratory problems;
- diabetes;
- digestive disorders;
- obesity;
- musculoskeletal diseases;
- cancer — lung, colorectal and breast cancer;
- viral infections.

It is also important to recognise that physical ill health can lead to a mental health problem. It is not uncommon for enduring physical health problems to be co-morbid with depression. These health problems include:

- cancer;
- heart disease;
- diabetes;
- musculoskeletal;
- respiratory problems.

Professional skills

Mental health nurses should:

- promote physical health and well-being through education, role modelling and effective communication;
- deliver physical care that meets the essential needs of people with mental health problems;
- recognise and respond to the physical needs of all individuals who come into their care;
- be able, where required, to signpost an individual with physical and mental health problems to the appropriate service.

Factors

There are numerous factors that might account for a higher incidence of physical ill health in individuals with mental health problems. These factors include:

- psychiatric medication — some medications increase the risk of obesity, diabetes and cardiac problems;

- lifestyle — individuals with mental health problems have a higher rate of smoking, and drug and alcohol misuse; they also tend to eat less well and exercise less;
- social — indirect factors such as poverty, poor housing and unemployment may also have an adverse impact.

There are also protective factors that keep mental health service users physically well such as:

- supportive and nurturing social networks;
- employment;
- self-awareness and having a sense of hope;
- having a healthy lifestyle.

Physical health assessment
Even when these factors are taken into account, individuals with mental health problems are less likely to have their physical health needs recognised than the general population. On this basis, a physical health assessment should include:

- the gathering of baseline physical health, including a medical history;
- a physical examination including baseline observations;
- baseline investigations including blood tests.

After the initial assessment the individual should be monitored annually, usually via their general practitioner (GP).

Managing physical health
The role of the mental health nurse in managing an individual's physical health is to be a health promoter, which includes:

- providing education about medication, including side effects;
- providing dietary advice or signposting to a dietician;
- promoting the benefits of physical exercise and monitoring weight;
- providing smoking cessation advice;
- liaising with the GP when required;
- signposting to family planning and sexual health services when required.

A key part of health promotion is to work collaboratively with the individual to change unhealthy behaviours by:

- recognising what behaviour needs to change;
- developing an agreed action plan;
- implementing the action plan;
- providing encouragement no matter how small the change;
- monitoring outcomes;
- developing agreed strategies to maintain change;
- persevering if the change does not happen.

Psychiatric examination

Background

The psychiatric examination is an assessment process carried out by a psychiatrist. The focus of the examination is to establish a diagnosis, formulate the problem (summarise the psychiatric examination), and then to provide a treatment plan. This process conceptualises the service user's mental distress through the lens of a medical diagnosis, so hearing voices and not coping from day-to-day can become a diagnosis of schizophrenia. This approach can be viewed as reductionist, whereby mental distress is reduced to a diagnosis and somehow the person suffering with the problem becomes forgotten. This does not have to be the case, however, as not all psychiatrists take a reductionist approach and, in addition, modern psychiatry is situated within a multidisciplinary team approach which, to function effectively, has to be holistic rather than reductionist.

The data gathered from the psychiatric examination, including the service user's history and information related to the presenting problem, feeds into the data collected by the multidisciplinary team. The mental health nurse will use this collective information in conjunction with the data they have collected through the care-planning process. The service user usually provides most of this information; however other parties may also be able to contribute, such as relatives and health and social care staff. This process has two distinct parts:

- the psychiatric history and mental state examination;
- the formulation.

Professional skills

Mental health nurses should:

- recognise different forms of mental distress and respond effectively, irrespective of age or setting, as part of a multidisciplinary team approach;
- have an in-depth understanding of the care and treatment of individuals with mental health needs;
- work within the context of a multidisciplinary team to enhance the care and treatment of individuals with mental health needs;
- apply and value the use of evidence within their practice and in their role as a member of a multidisciplinary team.

Psychiatric history

Physical examinations and investigations are carried out as part of the psychiatric examination more to exclude an underlying physical cause rather than to confirm a diagnosis. The psychiatry history is a catch-all term for the collection of a large amount of historical data. The information collected is structured through the following headings:

- introductory information — including age, occupation, reason for referral and status according to the *Mental Health Act 1983 (amended 2007)*;
- presenting complaint and history — including the service user's view of what the problem is, and identifying the nature of the service user's symptoms;
- past psychiatric history — including previous episodes of mental distress, the date of these episodes, the duration and any treatments;
- past medical history — including current and past physical illnesses and any subsequent treatments;
- drug history/current treatments — including psychosocial treatments, prescribed medication and allergies;
- substance abuse — including alcohol, illicit drugs and tobacco;
- family history — including any family history of mental health problems and any recent issues within the family;
- social history — including accommodation, finances, hobbies and activities;
- personal history — including childhood, education, employment history and forensic history;
- informant history — supplementing the service user's information with information from a significant alternative source, such as a relative.

The mental state examination
Complementing the psychiatric history, the mental state examination is a snapshot of the service user's behaviour and mental experiences at the time of the examination. It is usually structured using the following headings:

- appearance and behaviour;
- speech;
- mood — this would include asking about suicidal ideas;
- thoughts;
- perception;
- cognition;
- insight.

The formulation
The formulation summarises the whole psychiatric examination process and is structured using the following headings:

- synopsis;
- differential diagnosis;
- aetiology;
- investigations;

- management;
- prognosis.

Psychological interventions

Background

Mental health nursing practice should be holistic and mental health nurses are professionally required to have the skills, knowledge and values to deliver holistic care that is safe and effective. Psychological interventions are a crucial part of this holistic approach, especially as they aim to improve an individual's biopsychosocial functioning.

There is an increasing need for mental health nurses to be able to deliver psychological interventions as part of their everyday nursing practice. Clinical guidance related to specific mental disorders might recommend a specific psychological therapy and/or a number of psychological interventions — collectively known as 'psychosocial' interventions. In the wider context of mental health nursing practice psychological interventions are mental health nursing interventions underpinned by psychological methods and theory with the intention of improving biopsychosocial functioning. The delivery of physical healthcare interventions should also be supported by psychological theories and methods. Whatever the context, it is important to recognise that these interventions should be delivered through a therapeutically structured relationship built on good communication skills and a commitment to partnership working.

Professional skills

Mental health nurses should:

- use a wide range of therapeutic strategies and interventions, and communicate about these interventions effectively to optimise health and well-being;
- be person centred and committed to building therapeutic relationships that are enabling and partnership focused;
- deliver care across settings that is underpinned by a range of evidence-based psychological, psychosocial and other complex therapeutic skills and interventions;
- deliver care that is systematic, balances the need for safety with positive risk taking and promotes recovery.

Psychological therapies

The psychological therapies commonly used in mental health care include:

- cognitive behavioural therapies;
- cognitive stimulation;
- dialectic behaviour therapy;

- interpersonal therapy;
- motivational enhancement therapy;
- psychodynamic therapy;
- systemic family therapy.

Communication skills

Any psychological intervention or therapy should be built on good and effective communication skills. Being an effective communicator also means being a safe practitioner: someone who is ethical, engenders trust and openness, and builds therapeutic relationships that are collaborative and positive especially when managing risk.

Psychological interventions

Although psychological interventions are usually eclectic and may correspond to more than one psychological therapy or theory they still need to be delivered systematically in such a way that their effectiveness can be evaluated. Depending on the skill of the mental health nurse the following types of psychological interventions might be delivered:

- build a collaborative and therapeutic relationship based on a person-centred approach;
- normalise an individual's experiences of mental distress;
- take a 'strengths approach';
- maintain safety and manage challenging behaviours effectively;
- explore the individual's capacity to change;
- modify thought processes — identify, challenge and replace negative thoughts;
- focus on the individual controlling and regulating their behaviour — promote and enhance healthy ways of coping;
- prevent social isolation and promote social functioning;
- focus on relapse prevention — establishing early warning signs and self-monitoring of symptoms;
- signpost the individual to self-help and relevant support groups;
- support recovery therapeutically.

Psychological interventions should be:

- based on robust evidence;
- collaborative;
- embedded within the multiprofessional team;
- recovery focused;
- skilful.

Being evidence based

Mental health nurses should deliver psychological interventions that are based on the best evidence available. It is also important to recognise that generalised evidence needs to be situated within the unique nature of the therapeutic relationship. To do this the mental health nurse needs to complement the evidence-based knowledge with knowledge of the mental health service user they are working with. This comes from the use of good communication skills that focus on truly listening to the mental health service user's story.

Collaboration

Managing risk is an important part of the mental health nurse's role and being collaborative in this context can be a challenge, especially when the mental health nurse has the power to restrict the freedoms of a mental health service user. This type of power could have an adverse impact upon the therapeutic relationship and any subsequent psychological interventions that are delivered if it is not managed sensitively. To address both this power issue and also to continually improve their practice the mental health nurse must actively engage in critical reflection. The process of critical reflection starts with the mental health nurse using an 'open dialogue' approach that focuses on understanding and respecting the service user as a human being rather than as someone to be controlled. The next step is to learn from this approach through structured reflection such as participating in clinical supervision.

Psychological therapies

Background

On a day-to-day basis mental health nurses deliver psychological interventions; some of these interventions are clearly underpinned by a specific psychological approach or therapy. In fact, most psychological interventions delivered by mental health nurses will link to a corresponding psychological theory or model; however, due to the eclectic nature of mental health nursing it may be difficult to identify a specific supporting model or theory. To add further complexity the terms psychological interventions, psychosocial interventions, psychological therapies and psychotherapy are used interchangeably.

Psychological therapies are built on a platform of psychological interventions that are underpinned by a specific psychological model. For example, distraction as a psychological intervention would be used to deal with intrusive thoughts, which is a cognitive behavioural model, and the corresponding psychological therapy is cognitive behavioural therapy (CBT). Psychosocial interventions are psychological interventions which have a 'social' element such as an emphasis on social skills training and/or family interventions. Psychological therapies and psychotherapy can be viewed as synonymous and will sometimes be called 'talking therapies'. All mental health nurses should be able to deliver a number of different types of psychological interventions, though not all will be trained to deliver a specific psychological therapy.

Professional skills

Mental health nurses should:

- communicate effectively using a wide range of therapeutic strategies and interventions to optimise health, well-being and safety;
- use a range of evidence-based psychological, psychosocial and other complex therapeutic skills and interventions to provide person-centred care;
- deliver care across settings that is underpinned by a range of evidence-based psychological, psychosocial and other complex therapeutic skills and interventions;
- carry out systematic needs assessments, develop case formulations, negotiate goals and deliver both individual psychosocial interventions and group psychosocial interventions.

Behavioural therapy

Behavioural therapy focuses on behavioural change to influence the way we feel and act. For example, an individual might be fearful about specific situations to the point that they avoid this situation due to their overwhelming anxiety. Slowly learning to relax, even when they are exposed to this situation, can help them to both control their anxious feelings and stop using avoidant behaviours.

Cognitive therapy

Cognitive therapy is a short-term therapy concerned with modifying the way we think and then act. An individual might feel worthless, and use examples from their life to support this way of thinking. The mental health nurse challenges this way of thinking by supporting the individual to recognise what they can do rather than what they think they cannot.

Cognitive behavioural therapy

CBT is a short-term therapy that has components of both behavioural therapy and cognitive therapy. It focuses on changing both thinking and behaviour at the same time. It is recommended in the treatment of:

- depression;
- anxiety;
- obsessive compulsive disorder;
- post-traumatic stress disorder;
- eating disorders;
- psychosis.

CBT is available as a computerised package, and it can also be a component of other therapies, such as mindfulness-based cognitive therapy, dialectical behavioural therapy, and acceptance and commitment therapy.

Eye movement desensitisation and reprocessing

Eye movement desensitisation and reprocessing is a treatment that uses eye movements, sounds or taps to stimulate the way the brain processes information during an unpleasant memory such as those experienced during post-traumatic stress disorder. The underpinning theory is that the brain as an information processor becomes 'frozen' when an unpleasant memory is recalled, and by stimulating the brain when recalling the memory, the experience over time becomes less intense and has less of an impact upon the individual's ability to function.

Group therapy

Group therapy is an approach that utilises the psychological processes of the group to find facilitated solutions. This approach is based on the premise that the group has a dynamic that, if facilitated appropriately, is a safe way of motivating and supporting group members to become more aware about themselves and the way they function. By becoming more self-aware an individual is more likely to use healthier ways of coping.

Humanistic counselling

Humanistic counselling has a number of components; in essence, however, it is used to facilitate individuals to focus on their strengths to overcome their presenting mental distress. The approach is person centred meaning it values the person and their innate ability to find a solution.

Mindfulness-based therapies

Mindfulness-based therapies assist an individual to be in the moment, not to be overwhelmed by their mental distress, through techniques that are based on the principles of meditation. This approach can be combined with other therapies such as cognitive behavioural therapy.

Systemic therapy

Systemic therapy, which is also known as family therapy, focuses on managing and resolving an individual's mental distress through working with the interactions, patterns and dynamics of the individual's social group. The aim is to facilitate new, healthier interactions, patterns and dynamics to emerge.

Solution-focused therapy

Solution-focused therapy is also known as a brief therapy and it focuses, as the name suggests, on solutions rather than problems. The approach is goal focused; the individual identifies a goal and is then facilitated to achieve this goal by using their internal resources, and/or developing new resources and/or using the resources of their social network.

Recovery

Background

Recovery as a therapeutic process is an integral part of mental health nursing practice. As a process, mental health nurses often see recovery in terms of eliminating or controlling symptoms of mental distress. This view is quite a narrow, as recovery should be a whole-person approach whereby the meaning of recovery is embedded within the hopes and aspirations of the individual. Recovery is also about social inclusion, whereby individuals are supported to live meaningful lives within society.

Utilising a recovery-based approach presents a significant challenge for mental health nurses especially when there are professional and policy drivers that require mental health nurses to utilise a recovery-based approach but at the same time there is no single agreed definition of recovery. With this in mind, recovery should be viewed relative to the individual and their circumstances, meaning that the recovery process for that individual is constantly redefined by their ever-changing needs. The challenge for the mental health nurse in these circumstances is that they need to be both receptive and responsive to the service user's ever-evolving needs and ensure that their practice is positively redefined by these experiences. Even though recovery as process is relative in nature it can have aims which include:

- promoting well-being;
- maximising opportunity;
- empowering individuals to take control;
- facilitating and supporting the individual in finding meaning and purpose.

Professional skills

Mental health nurses should:

- engage effectively with individuals with mental health problems in a way that is person centred and also promotes social inclusion and recovery;
- ensure their practice is recovery focused whatever the context or setting, and that it values, respects and explores the meaning of an individual's mental distress;
- promote the self-determination expertise of individuals with mental health problems while using their personal qualities and interpersonal skills to develop and maintain a recovery-focused therapeutic relationship;
- work with people living with mental distress and with other professionals and agencies to shape services in a way that aids recovery.

The recovery process

Recovery can be described in terms of a process which includes the following features:

- a whole-person approach is taken rather than just focusing on symptoms;
- recovery is viewed as a journey rather than a destination;
- optimism, commitment and hope are key values;
- support should be systematic but also innovative.

The components of recovery

There are a number of models of recovery, including the:

- Collaborative Recovery Model
- Strengths Model
- Tidal Model
- Well-being and Recovery Action Plan Approach

The Tidal Model is particularly pertinent to mental health nurses as it was created by mental health nurses in collaboration with mental health service users. The Tidal Model is made up of three key components or domains:

- self domain — narrative or story-telling component;
- world domain — the narrative component is shared with others;
- others domain — recovery is enacted through the care-delivery process.

Policy

Recovery is a key objective within the *No Health without Mental Health* policy document (DoH 2011a), which focuses on good quality care for people with:

- emerging mental health problems;
- acute mental distress;
- ongoing mental health problems.

Integrating the recovery approach within the care-delivery process should help:

- reduce distress;
- improved social functioning;
- maintain and develop good relationships;
- provide the opportunity for education, skills, employment and purpose;
- maintain good physical health;
- reduce the risk of relapse.

The recovery approach

During the recovery process the mental health nurse must be able to support the individual such that the individual's story is actively valued as a core part of the care-delivery process. The nurse must also recognise that interventions have to be outcome focused and adaptable to changing need. Building on this, the nurse must also be aware of the factors that influence the recovery process positively, including:

- positive and sustainable relationships;
- paid employment;
- meaningful activity;
- autonomy;
- resilience;
- personal growth;
- a healthy living environment;
- a supportive social network.

Reflection

Background

Mental health nurses are professionally required to engage in the process of reflection, the most common form of which is 'reflection on action', which involves reflecting on practice experiences in a way that promotes learning. For this process to be effective the nurse needs to be committed to better understanding their own values and how these relate to the values of the nursing profession; they also need to be committed to improving their practice constantly. A common method of systematically reflecting on practice is through clinical supervision, which is a formal activity whereby a clinical supervisor facilitates the nurse to reflect upon their practice and identify strategies that focus on improving their practice.

The professional expectation is that at the point of registration the mental health nurse is a critically reflective practitioner who learns from practice in a way that improves the quality of the care they deliver. Being critically reflective implies that the nurse is able to identify critical incidents that arise from their practice experiences. This essentially a process of questioning during which the nurse should consider:

- What is the issue, is it problematic and why?
- Why has it occurred?
- How does this issue impact upon the service user?
- What are the options or alternatives?
- Have you looked at the evidence?

The skills of critical reflection arise from engaging in reflection in two interconnected forms:

- reflection on action — reflecting after an experience and then taking action to improve practice;
- reflection in action — reflecting during the experience so that previous learning can be used to improve practice at that moment in time.

Professional skills
Mental health nurses should:

- participate actively in clinical supervision and reflection;
- engage in reflection and supervision to ensure they learn from their practice experiences in a way that enhances the quality of care they provide;
- participate in the reflective process as a mechanism to better understand their personal values, beliefs and emotions and how they can impact upon their practice;
- actively promote clinical supervision as clinical leader and as clinical role model.

Structured reflection
For reflection to be useful or action focused it has to have a structured process. A number of models are available and most have a common structure, such as:

- identifying and describing the experience/s;
- examining the experience in depth, teasing out the key issues: What did I think at the time? How did I feel?
- processing the issues: How do the issues relate to practice? What have I learnt?
- summarising the experience: What actions do I need to take? How can I improve my practice?

Learning to reflect in a structured way is important but it should not be used as rigid formula, instead it should be used as a guide. It is also important to recognise that reflection on action, if used properly as a lifelong learning tool, will become more refined over time; it will also enable the nurse to reflect in action and assist them towards being an expert practitioner.

Clinical supervision
Clinical supervision as a reflective practice can be delivered in different ways, including:

- individual supervision;
- group supervision;
- peer group supervision.

Although clinical supervision follows the tenets of structured reflection it can be grounded in a specific model, especially when a mental health nurse is also a therapist, such as a cognitive behavioural therapist. Whichever model is used in clinical supervision, as a professional process it should:

- support practice and enable the nurse to maintain and promote standards of care;
- be a practice-focused professional relationship, involving a practitioner reflecting on practice guided by a skilled supervisor;
- be developed by practitioners and managers according to local circumstances; ground rules should be agreed so that practitioners and supervisors approach clinical supervision openly and confidently, and are aware of what is involved;
- ensure that all practitioners should have access to clinical supervision and each supervisor should supervise a realistic number of practitioners;
- ensure supervisors are adequately prepared with the principles and relevance of clinical supervision that is included in pre- and post-registration education programmes;
- be evaluated locally with a focus on evaluating how clinical supervision influences care, practice standards and the mental health service.

Lifelong learning
To have real value, lifelong learning (which includes continuing professional development) has to have a reflective component. Nurses who are lifelong learners and critically reflective are capable practitioners who:

- know how to learn and reflect continually;
- work well with others and are effective communicators;
- regularly and easily apply themselves to new and unfamiliar situations;
- demonstrate positive values about themselves and others.

Research

Background
Utilising good quality research evidence will assist the mental health nurse in the process of providing a continuous high standard of care with improved care outcomes. To utilise such evidence effectively and appropriately the nurse will need to be competent in the use of research-based evidence. Part of being competent is knowing what evidence is useful and what evidence is not so useful, and also being able to justify the decision taken. It is worth noting that there are

different forms of knowledge, but, in terms of clinical guidelines, scientific evidence is the key form of knowledge used in mental health nursing practice.

Nursing practice utilises different types of knowledge:

- traditional and routine-based knowledge;
- experienced-based knowledge;
- research-based knowledge.

The nurse will not use one source of knowledge exclusively; as an example, research might suggest the nurse should change their practice in a certain way and experience may further modify this change, which then becomes the norm or traditional practice. Research is a systematic way of gaining knowledge where what is already known is either added to, rejected or confirmed. It can assist the nurse in the process of:

- exploring the issues in further depth;
- solving problems;
- providing a strong rationale for change.

Research is generally either quantitative, focusing on measuring cause and effect, or qualitative, which is more concerned with value-laden or subjective issues.

Professional skills

Mental health nurses should:

- deliver care that is responsive to the needs of individuals living with mental health problems and is based appropriately on research evidence;
- ensure their practice is informed by the best available evidence and complies with local and national guidelines;
- recognise the value of evidence in practice and be able to understand and appraise research, apply relevant theory and research findings to practice, and identify areas for further investigation;
- use research-based evidence to assist in improving improve mental health service users care experiences and care outcomes and also to shape future care provision.

Scientific evidence

Scientific evidence (also called quantitative evidence) and approaches take different forms, though the dominate form in mental health nursing practice is the evidence-based form or what is called evidence-based practice (EBP). This means that the clinical-decision-making process is based on the careful use of current and best available evidence. This evidence can range from testimony from a clinical expert to evidence that is collected through randomised controlled trials (RCTs). The highest quality evidence is collected through the RCT process. It is important to note that this type of evidence is continually being updated and, on this basis, the nurse needs to ensure they too are regularly updated about any changes. This should include checking any relevant clinical guidelines that are based upon EBP, as the guidelines change as the evidence is updated. EBP has number of steps, starting with asking a clinical question such as; What is the best nursing intervention for this condition? The nurse will then move on to:

- identifying the relevant literature;
- assessing the evidence critically; Is it reliable and/or valid?
- applying the chosen evidence to the particular clinical situation;
- evaluating the application of the evidence.

Naturalistic evidence

Naturalistic research (also called qualitative research) investigates experiences and meanings, such as why individuals act in the way they do. The different types of naturalistic research approaches include:

- phenomenology;
- grounded theory;
- ethnography;
- narrative studies;
- case studies.

The most commonly used methods of collecting information for these approaches are:

- interviews;
- narratives;
- case studies;
- focus groups.

Practice evidence

EBP is a dominant approach, although it is important to recognise that scientific knowledge only provides one perspective, which can be a limited way of understanding a service user's mental distress. A better understanding can be engendered through multiple approaches, which might include working with both EBP information and the service user's narrative. By working in this manner, with both scientific and naturalistic knowledge, the nurse has a more holistic understanding of a mental health service user's needs. When working with a service user's narrative or story it is important that the nurse really listens and pays attention to the purpose, content and tone of the story:

- purpose — what information is contained within the narrative and why is the service user giving you this information?
- content — what does the narrative say about the service user's quality of life?
- tone — is the overall tone positive or negative?

Suicide and self-harm

Background

Managing suicide and self-harm are part of managing risk. The risk-management process should be partnership focused and emotionally intelligent, as the emotions related to harm, whether it be harm to self or others, can be intense and distressing. The mental health nurse also has to recognise that the levels of risk attributed to suicide and self-harm can change quite quickly, and when risk levels increase a service user's freedoms may be restricted which, in itself, can be distressing.

Suicide is a form of self-harm; however, individuals may engage in acts of deliberate self-harm with no intention of committing suicide. It is important to note that individuals who engage in deliberate self-harm are more likely to commit suicide than the general population (Burton 2006). Suicide and self-harm can be categorised as follows:

- suicide — intentionally killing oneself;
- attempted suicide — intentionally trying to kill oneself without success;
- parasuicide — trying to kill oneself and not succeeding, it may or may not be intentional, it may be a suicidal gesture, a cry for help or an act of revenge;
- deliberate self-harm — intentionally injuring oneself; there may or may not be suicidal intent. Acts that have little or no suicidal intent may be a way of coping with emotional and mental distress or a way of communicating distress.

Professional skills

Mental health nurses should:

- recognise and manage suicide and self-harm in a way that is person centred, recovery focused and that protects vulnerable individuals;
- work positively and proactively with individuals who are at risk of suicide and self-harm, using evidence-based models of suicide prevention, intervention and harm reduction to prevent, reduce and minimise the risk;

- manage the risk of suicide and self-harm both independently and as part of a team approach in a way that promotes effective communication, positive risk management and continuity of care across services;
- respond autonomously and appropriately when faced with self-harm and attempted suicide, including seeking help from appropriate individuals when necessary.

Suicide

Since 1961 suicide has been decriminalised in the UK; however the act of assisting someone to commit suicide is still illegal. In other cultures suicide can be viewed as an honourable death in certain circumstances, in the UK, however, the sanctity of life argument holds sway. It is estimated that that the majority of suicides can be linked to a mental disorder such as:

- depression;
- substance misuse;
- personality disorder;
- psychosis.

Suicide is the fourth commonest cause of death in the UK, and it is thought that published suicide rates do not reflect the fact that suicides may well be under-reported. Risk factors for suicide include:

- gender — men are three times more likely to commit suicide than women;
- age — the highest suicide rates are for men between 25 and 45 years old and women over 65 years old;
- whether single, widowed or separated/divorced;
- whether unemployed or retired;
- certain occupations — vets, farmers, pharmacists and doctors;
- social isolation;
- whether a victim of physical or sexual abuse;
- a recent life crisis;
- a history of deliberate self-harm;
- a mental disorder;
- a severe physical illness;
- a family history of suicide or deliberate self-harm.

Hanging is the most common method of suicide for men and poisoning is the most common method for women.

Self-harm

Accurate rates of deliberate self-harm are difficult to ascertain as not everyone who deliberately self-harms will go to hospital or seek medical attention. Within England and Wales it is estimated that there are at least 200,000 hospital admissions or presentations per year for deliberate self-harm. Self-poisoning and self-injury by cutting are the most common types of deliberate self-harm. Risk factors include:

- age — deliberate self-harm is more common in people under the age of 25;
- gender — deliberate self-harm is more common in women than men;
- a mental disorder;
- substance misuse;
- whether a victim of physical or sexual abuse;
- relationship changes;
- social isolation;
- bereavement;
- unemployment.

Management
When a service user attempts suicide within a mental health ward it is important that staff have the appropriate life-support training and that the equipment is checked regularly and is up-to-date. As this is a medical emergency the paramedics also need to be contacted. When a service user engages in deliberate self-harm the mental health nurse should:

- establish the likely physical risk to themselves and to others;
- de-escalate and control the incident;
- assess the extent of the injury;
- refer the service user for urgent treatment in an emergency department if required;
- provide treatment as required in a respectful and person-centred manner.

Assessment
The assessment of service users who have self-harmed should be part of the risk-assessment process. The following areas should be assessed as part of this process:

- skills, strengths and assets of the service user;
- coping strategies;
- mental health problems;
- physical health problems;
- social circumstances and problems;
- methods and frequency of current and past self-harm;
- current and past suicidal intent;
- depressive symptoms and their relationship to self-harm;
- triggers, specific risk factors and protective factors;
- significant relationships;
- immediate and long-term risks.

Psychological interventions

In the short term the mental health nurse should consider using psychological interventions that help reduce harm, which include:

- reinforcing existing coping strategies that are healthy;
- supporting the service user to develop less harmful ways of coping;
- supporting the service user to develop effective problem-solving skills;
- advising the service user that there is no safe way to self-poison.

In the long term the service user should be offered a psychological therapy; the type of therapy will depend on whether the self-harm co-exists with an underlying mental health condition.

Therapeutic relationships

Background

Therapeutic relationships in mental health nursing should be evidence based, especially when delivering psychological interventions, and they should also respect the narrative of the service user. Mental health nurses are therefore required to build a therapeutic relationship that acknowledges the service user's unique narrative and at the same time delivers positive therapeutic outcomes. The therapeutic use of self is crucial within the process of developing meaningful and positive therapeutic relationships. It is also important to note that the use of self in a recovery-based relationship needs to be underpinned by the mental health nurse's commitment to partnership working.

At times it can become quite easy for the mental health nurse to reconstruct the service user's own experience of mental distress. This can happen for example when an assessment tool is being used which captures the information the mental health nurse needs; however it does not capture the service user's entire story. Having different viewpoints can create conflict within the relationship unless the mental health nurse takes a collaborative approach. In addition, the therapeutic relationship within the mental health field has an element of risk when, for example, risk containment and risk minimisation shape the relationship. Even though the therapeutic relationship is intended to be collaborative and person centred this intention is dependent on the level of risk. The nurse should always look to build therapeutic relationships that are based on true partnership working and, at the same time, value both the service user and their experiences; a person-centred philosophy.

Professional skills

Mental health nurses should:

- build safe therapeutic relationships that are partnership focused, person centred and non-discriminatory;
- use relationship-building skills with mental health service users, including facilitating therapeutic groups;

- use their personal qualities, experiences and interpersonal skills to build recovery-focused relationships;
- be self-aware and know to when to use self-disclosure while maintaining professional boundaries;
- recognise mental distress and be able to respond using therapeutic principles that are underpinned by evidence-based practice.

The therapeutic self
Mental health nurses use a range of strategies in the process of building a therapeutic relationship. These strategies include:

- selecting the right words to use;
- knowing when to talk and when to be silent;
- using the right verbal and non-verbal responses;
- adapting non-verbal communication to suit the situation.

To use these strategies effectively the mental health nurse needs to be self-aware; aware of the impact their self has upon others, and aware of their own thoughts and feelings. They also need to be able to use this knowledge in a positive way when working with service users.

Empathy
It is essential that the mental health nurse is empathetic within the therapeutic relationship. This means that they have to be able to identify with the service user's experiences by being:

- an active listener;
- genuinely interested;
- accepting the person;
- caring and compassionate.

Delivering care
The *No Health without Mental Health* policy document (DoH 2011a) and its accompanying strategy and vision document for mental health nursing (DoH 2011b) highlight the importance of partnership working. The vision document links explicitly to the 6Cs, and within the 'care' element the development of a sustainable and positive therapeutic relationship is viewed as the basis for all the care that the mental health nurse provides. This relationship needs to be:

- grounded in compassion;
- respectful and empathetic;
- skilful and purposeful;
- recovery focused and inclusive.

Professional boundaries
Taking an empathetic approach gives the nurse the opportunity to be more thoughtful about the interventions they deliver, but also on occasion the nurse may self-disclose. As a therapeutic skill

self- disclosure can be a way of fostering collaboration. When using self-disclosure the mental health nurse must remember that, as a nursing professional, there are professional boundaries that they must adhere to in addition to being governed by a professional code of conduct.

Reflective practice

To build therapeutic relationships that have positive outcomes the mental health nurse needs to be able to balance being person centred and collaborative against the demands of being a clinical risk manager. To do this effectively the mental health nurse has to be able to engage in reflective practice, which is a professional requirement as well as an important component of effective clinical decision-making. Reflective practice is a structured and critical process that requires the nurse to re-examine their practice experiences and focus on changing their practice for the better.

Time management

Background

When in the process of delivering care, mental health nurses have to manage their time effectively. Time management is a complex process; it is concerned not only with how the mental health nurse manages their own time as a series of tasks, but also how they manage time pressure emotionally. A nurse who is an expert in a certain intervention may take less time to complete it than someone who is less experienced. This in itself is not problematic; the problem arises if the team expectation is that everyone can complete the intervention in the same amount of time. If a nurse cannot meet this expectation they can feel rushed or they rush to complete the intervention and consequently feel stressed. Another issue is that the delivery of mental health nursing care can be routine focused with tasks planned in advance, but the routine has to be flexible as unexpected issues can arise which have to be dealt with immediately.

Care delivery has become increasingly complex and the mental nurse needs to manage many competing priorities. Managing time focuses on controlling the amount of time and effort spent on a specific task or intervention, including:

- prioritising tasks;
- scheduling the order of tasks to be undertaken;
- planning each task;
- agreeing what needs to be achieved;
- allocating resources to the task;
- delegating when required.

Being systematic can be extremely helpful in managing time but, as health and social care provision can change rapidly, it is important that this approach is flexible. Prioritisation should be the mediating factor in a flexible approach; for example, writing a care plan might well be a priority before an emergency situation arises on the ward, and then the emergency takes priority. On this basis mental health nurse should:

- be aware of what are priorities and what are not;
- set priorities being aware that they can change;
- deliver care based on those priorities.

Professional skills
Mental health nurses should:

- identify priorities and manage time and resources effectively to ensure that the quality of care is maintained or enhanced;
- prioritise the needs of groups and individuals in order to provide care effectively and efficiently;
- negotiate with others in relation to balancing competing and conflicting priorities;
- prioritise own workload and manage competing and conflicting priorities.

Delegation
When a team is delivering care then tasks need to be allocated, and the person undertaking the task should be the best person for the job. In an ideal situation the team would allocate their own tasks, but usually task allocation falls to the team leader. The appropriate and safe use of delegation can create a sense of time and space; one person does not feel they are doing everything. When delegating tasks the following should be considered:

- Does the person have the right skills and knowledge?
- Are they legally allowed to undertake the task?
- What does the organisation's policy say?
- Who is accountable and responsible?
- Does the person know exactly what they need to do?
- Is delegating the task the best option?

Stress management
The benefit of being a good time manager is that it helps the mental health nurse cope with stress in a healthy way. Stress in itself is not a bad thing; it is usually transient, and at times we all feel a bit stressed. It becomes problematic, however, when the mental or emotional pressure adversely impacts upon an individual's ability to function healthily; in other words an individual may feel unable to cope. People have different stress levels and different ways of coping; it is therefore important for mental health nurses to recognise when they are

stressed and whether stress is having a negative impact upon their ability to cope. Prolonged stress manifests different ways, including:

- sleep problems;
- loss of appetite;
- difficulty concentrating;
- constantly feeling anxious;
- feeing irritable and/or angry;
- having repeating thoughts;
- worrying;
- avoiding certain situations and/or people;
- an increased use of alcohol;
- headaches;
- muscle tension.

Prolonged stress can lead to the individual experiencing emotional exhaustion and, in some cases, leading to a number of mental disorders. To manage stress consider the following activities:

- engage in physical activity;
- engage in something that makes you laugh;
- learn relaxation and/or deep breathing techniques;
- take control of the situation;
- seek support and talk;
- try to find a solution to the problem;
- eat a healthily diet;
- drink plenty of water;
- be mindful.

Values-based practice

Background

All nurses are required to practice ethically, which includes being able to reason ethically. The added dimension for mental health nurses is that they have to also take into account the value-laden nature of mental health practice.

The mental health nurse must know how to act ethically and they must also be able to justify their actions. The need to act ethically is also contextualised by the controlling element of mental health nursing practice whereby the mental health nurse might have the power to restrict a service user's freedoms in some cases. Where there is the power to restrict freedoms there is potential for ethical conflict; for example, a mental health nurse might justify this power on the basis that they are keeping the service user safe, whereas the service user might see this power in a more negative light, as an abuse of power. Where this conflict arises and different values are at play within the therapeutic relationship the conflict needs to be managed in way that is collaborative and recovery focused.

Professional skills

Mental health nurses should:

- be able to understand the importance of values and beliefs and how they impact upon the communication process;
- work within recognised professional, ethical and legal frameworks;
- ensure that decisions about care are shared and in a way that values a service user's experiences;
- recognise and address ethical and legal challenges that arise within the therapeutic relationship.

Ethical theory

In general, ethical theories that influence mental health nursing practice are normative, focusing on what actions are right, what ought to be done, which motives are good, and which characteristics are virtuous; for example:

- consequentialism (also known as utilitarianism) is outcome focused; for the mental health nurse to be ethical their actions need to produce the greatest balance of good over bad;
- deontology (also known as Kantianism) is concerned with duty; without exception the ethical mental health nurse must always do their ethical/professional duty;
- virtue ethics are based on the character of a person; a virtuous mental health nurse will acquire and utilise virtuous traits such as honesty, trustworthiness, cooperativeness and humility;
- principlism is using principles in ethical decision-making, such as do no harm (non-maleficence), act to benefit others (beneficence), respect a person's autonomy and treat people fairly (justice).

Code of conduct

The Nursing & Midwifery Council in the UK requires mental health nurses to follow a professional code of conduct, which is based on four main ethical statements and twenty-five sub-statements (NMC 2015):

- prioritise people;
  - treat people as individuals and uphold their dignity;
  - listen to people and respond to their preferences and concerns;
  - act in the best interests of people at all times;
  - respect people's right to privacy and confidentiality;
- practise effectively;
  - always practise in line with the best available evidence;
  - communicate clearly;
  - work cooperatively;
  - share your skills, knowledge and experience for the benefit of people receiving care and your colleagues;

- keep clear and accurate records relevant to your practice;
- be accountable for your decisions to delegate tasks and duties to other people;
- have in place an indemnity arrangement which provides appropriate cover for any practice you take on as a nurse or midwife in the united kingdom;
- preserve safety;
  - recognise and work within the limits of your competence;
  - be open and candid with all service users about all aspects of care and treatment, including when any mistakes or harm have taken place;
  - always offer help if an emergency arises in your practice setting or anywhere else;
  - act without delay if you believe that there is a risk to patient safety or public protection;
  - raise concerns immediately if you believe a person is vulnerable or at risk and needs extra support and protection;
  - advise on, prescribe, supply, dispense or administer medicines within the limits of your training and competence, the law, our guidance and other relevant policies, guidance and regulations;
  - be aware of, and reduce as far as possible, any potential for harm associated with your practice;
- promote professionalism and trust;
  - uphold the reputation of your profession at all times;
  - uphold your position as a registered nurse or midwife;
  - fulfil all registration requirements;
  - cooperate with all investigations and audits;
  - respond to any complaints made against you professionally;
  - provide leadership to make sure people's well-being is protected and to improve their experiences of the healthcare system.

Ethical reasoning

Ethical theories and the NMC code of conduct should underpin the mental health nurse's ethical reasoning, and using an ethical framework can further assist this process:

1. Recognise the ethical issue/s;
2. Gather the facts and values;
3. Consider the rules;
4. Look at any underpinning moral theories;
5. Consider all options;
6. Make a decision and test it;
7. Act and reflect on the outcome.

Values-based practice

When gathering facts as part of the ethical reasoning process the mental health nurse also needs to gather values. Values-based practice is a process that focuses on dealing with conflicting values rather than outcomes. This process requires the mental health nurse to work with values in a way that resolves ethical conflict and moves the therapeutic relationship forward:

- consider the service user's perspective;
- balance the rules against this perspective;
- preserve the person-centred element of this perspective;
- represent this perspective fully in the decision-making process.

Conditions

Rapid Mental Health Nursing, First Edition. Grahame Smith and Rebecca Rylance.
© 2016 John Wiley & Sons, Ltd. Published 2016 by John Wiley & Sons, Ltd.

Acute confusional state

Definition
An acute confusional state (also called delirium) is characterised by severe confusion that has a rapid onset; the intensity of the symptoms can also fluctuate. There is usually a physical cause such as:

- alcohol, opiates or prescribed medication;
- renal, hepatic or cardiac failure;
- an underlying infection;
- hypoglycaemia;
- stroke;
- postoperative states.

A diagnosis is made if the following are present:

- impaired consciousness and attention;
- perceptual or cognitive disturbances;
- sudden onset with fluctuating intensity;
- an identifiable cause.

Types
Depending on the presentation of these symptoms, acute confusional state can be subdivided into three types:

- hypoactive delirium — the service user is quiet and withdrawn;
- hyperactive delirium — the service user is restless and agitated;
- mixed — the service user displays both types of behaviours.

Clinical features
As a clinical syndrome acute confusional state can encompass a range of symptoms, including:

- impaired consciousness and attention;
- memory problems;
- disorientation;
- language disturbances;
- hallucinations;
- transient delusions;
- sleep disturbances;
- drowsiness;
- mood fluctuation;
- restlessness;
- apathy;
- sweating;
- tachycardia.

Risk factors

Acute confusional state can be difficult to diagnose as other conditions can present with the same symptoms, including:

- depression;
- mania;
- dementia;
- schizophrenia.

Around one-third of adults aged 65 or older and in hospital present with delirium either on admission or during their hospital stay. A number of risk factors can increase the risk of an individual developing the condition:

- if they are aged 65 or over;
- if they have been diagnosed with a dementia;
- if they have a current hip fracture;
- if they are severely physically ill.

Management

The management of acute confusional state focuses on the identification and treatment of the underlying cause. A number of investigations need to be carried out, including:

- a full and comprehensive history;
- a mental state assessment;
- a physical examination;
- blood tests;
- urine test;
- chest X-ray;
- brain imaging;
- electroencephalography.

When the cause is identified the underlying condition can be treated. Until the individual's acute confusional state is resolved treatment guidelines recommend the use of non-pharmacological interventions as the first option. Pharmacological interventions are recommended only when distress and/or risk is not being sufficiently managed by the use of non-pharmacological interventions.

Psychological interventions

As acute confusional state has an underlying physical cause most individuals with the condition will be nursed within an adult nursing environment, such as an acute medical ward. The mental health nurse's role in the management of delirium is preventative, which includes:

- building a therapeutic relationship;
- reducing disorientation;
- promoting physical well-being, including nutritional diet and physical activity;
- utilising verbal and non-verbal de-escalation techniques where required.

Alcohol misuse

Definition

Alcohol misuse occurs when an individual's alcohol use has a harmful impact, such as physical, social and psychological harms. The individual may or may not be dependent on alcohol; signs of dependency include:

- compulsion to take alcohol;
- an adverse impact upon the individual's social functioning;
- the individual is tolerant to alcohol;
- the individual has difficulty in controlling their alcohol use;
- stopping their alcohol use causes withdrawal symptoms.

Types

Alcohol use is usually described in terms of safe limits, which in the UK is defined as 21 units of alcohol per week for men and 14 units per week for women (a unit of alcohol is approximately a small glass of wine or half a pint of beer). Alcohol abuse can be divided into:

- hazardous drinking — men consume 22–50 units per week and women 15–35 units per week;
- harmful drinking — men consume over 50 units per week and women over 35 units per week;
- binge drinking — consuming double the weekly safe limit of units in one day.

Alcohol disorders include:

- intoxication;
- harmful alcohol use;
- dependence;
- withdrawal state.

Clinical features

Alcohol misuse can lead to:

- disturbed consciousness and perception;
- damage to an individual's health and social functioning;

- neglect;
- physical and psychological withdrawal;
- hallucinations and delusions;
- memory and cognitive impairments.

Risk factors

Approximately one-quarter of the UK population exceeds the safe limits for alcohol consumption (DoH 2007b). The causes of alcohol misuse are not clear, although there are a number of factors that increase an individual's risk:

- availability of alcohol;
- peer pressure;
- a co-morbid mental health disorder;
- stressful situations or circumstances;
- a family history of alcohol misuse;
- life events, including childhood abuse and loss.

Management

The management of alcohol misuse is dependent on the presentation; an individual can present with signs of acute intoxication, withdrawal or dependency. The assessment of the individual is extremely important as a head injury can present as acute alcohol intoxication. Treatment guidelines recommend:

- acute detoxification;
- motivational enhancement therapy;
- cognitive behavioural therapy;
- abstinence;
- social learning strategies;
- self-help groups.

Psychological interventions

It is important to note that the way an individual uses alcohol can change over time, and they may spontaneously stop their alcohol misuse. Service users who misuse alcohol are usually treated outside of the mental health inpatient setting; however, mental health nurses will encounter individuals who both misuse alcohol and have a co-morbid mental health disorder. After the detoxification phase the mental health nurse will need to deliver different types of psychological interventions, which include:

- building a collaborative and therapeutic relationship;
- motivational and brief intervention work;
- guided self-help;
- coping strategy work;

- health promotion;
- family and couples work;
- contingency approaches — using incentives to change behaviour.

Anxiety and related conditions

Definition
When we are anxious we might feel frightened and apprehensive; we might also feel physically tense with a sense that our heart is beating faster than normal. Anxiety becomes problematic when it interferes with our ability to function, which can happen when there are persistent and enduring feelings of dread, apprehension and uneasiness, even when there is no recognisable danger.

Types
Anxiety disorders can be divided into three main types:

- generalised anxiety disorder (GAD) — a generalised and persistent anxiety lasting longer than three weeks;
- panic disorder — recurrent and severe panic attacks that occur unpredictably (a minimum of three panic attacks over a three week period);
- phobia — a fear that can become panic when exposed to specific situations, for example, places, objects, animals, heights and closed or open spaces.

A related disorder is obsessive compulsive disorder, which is characterised by recurrent obsessional thoughts or compulsive acts with a frequency greater than one hour per day and with a duration of at least two weeks.

Clinical features
Individuals with an anxiety disorder can experience a range of cognitive, behavioural and physical symptoms, including:

- fear and worry;
- increased vigilance;
- irritability and restlessness;
- poor concentration;
- sleeping difficulties;
- physical tension;
- hyperactivity;
- palpitations;
- abdominal discomfit and nausea;
- hot flushes;
- outbursts of anger;
- ruminating thoughts and compulsions.

Risk factors

The prevalence of anxiety disorders in the general population in the UK is around 6% at any one time (Katona *et al.* 2012), with GAD being the most common anxiety disorder. There are a number of factors that increase an individual's risk of an anxiety:

- gender — the condition is more common in women;
- age — the condition is more common in younger and middle-aged adults;
- drug misuse can heightened anxiety states;
- a family history of anxiety or a related condition;
- life events, such as childhood abuse, loss of employment, parental loss, excessive demands or high expectations;
- severe physical illness.

Management

Anxiety disorders are usually treated within a primary-care setting following a stepped-care model. The specific interventions employed are dependent on both the condition and the individual's preference. Treatment guidelines recommend:

- cognitive behavioural therapy;
- behavioural therapy;
- medication, such as selective serotonin re-uptake inhibitors;
- interpersonal therapy;
- group therapy;
- psychodynamic therapy;
- mindfulness approaches;
- systemic therapy;
- eye movement desensitisation;
- relaxation techniques.

Psychological interventions

Mental health nurses will encounter individuals who have been diagnosed with an anxiety disorder either on its own or as a co-morbid disorder with, for example, depression, substance misuse or another anxiety disorder. In either case it is important that mental health nurses follow a stepped-care model that is designed to indicate the choice of intervention by the severity of the episode. Risk needs to be managed as part of the delivery of any psychological intervention as well as ensuring that an effective therapeutic relationship has been built with the service user. Depending on the skill and training of the nurse the interventions that can be delivered include:

- guided self-help;
- breathing and relaxation exercises;

- identifying, challenging and replacing negative thoughts;
- motivational interviewing;
- grade exposure and response prevention;
- desensitisation.

Bipolar affective disorder

Definition

Bipolar affective disorder, which is also historically known as manic depression, is classified as a psychosis. Bipolar affective disorder is a disorder whereby an individual fluctuates between low and high mood states, including;

- depressive episodes;
- manic episodes;
- hypomanic episodes;
- mixed episodes.

Types

Bipolar affective disorder can be categorised into different types as follows:

- bipolar I — one or more manic episodes;
- bipolar II — recurrent severe depression and hypomanic episodes;
- rapid cycling — more than four mood swings in a 12-month period;
- cyclothymia — enduring mood fluctuations that are not as severe as in the other three types.

Clinical features

The key feature of bipolar affective disorder is the fluctuation in mood states, especially the presence of mania (an elevated or high mood state) and, to a lesser degree, hypomania. Other features include:

- an inflated sense of self-esteem and grandiose ideas;
- a decreased need for sleep;
- talking rapidly with racing thoughts;
- being easily distracted and over-active;
- delusions and hallucinations — in mania only;
- engaging in risky behaviours.

Risk factors

It is estimated that around 4% of individuals will experience a bipolar affective disorder over a lifetime (Katona *et al*. 2012). Risk factors include:

- presence of a bipolar affective disorder amongst first-degree relatives;
- higher social class;

- life events, such as childhood abuse and loss;
- sleep problems;
- age — bipolar affective disorder is more prevalent in the early twenties;
- gender — bipolar II is more prevalent in women;
- severe physical illness, for example, stroke.

Management

The first-line treatment for bipolar affective disorder focuses on psychiatric medication that reduces the severity of the symptoms, stabilises mood fluctuation and prevents relapse. Due to the type of medications that are prescribed to treat bipolar affective disorder individuals who are being treated should also have an annual physical health review. Treatment guidelines also recommend:

- cognitive behavioural therapy;
- family-focused therapy;
- psychoeducation;
- interpersonal therapy;
- electroconvulsive therapy for severe mania or depression.

Psychological interventions

Individuals diagnosed with a bipolar affective disorder might require rapid access to support, especially when they are experiencing severe symptoms. Managing risk to self and/or others might be a priority, particularly when an individual's mood is elevated. In this case it is important to provide an environment that is low in stimulation, ensure that the individual's dietary and fluid needs are met and only use physical restraint as a last option; de-escalation techniques are always preferable. The mental health nurse will also need to:

- build a collaborative and therapeutic relationship;
- provide psychoeducation, including medication adherence information;
- signpost the service user to self-help and relevant support groups;
- undertake relapse work, including identifying early warning signs and self-monitoring of symptoms;
- undertake coping strategy work.

Child and adolescent mental health

Definition

Mental health problems in children and adolescents can be mild to severe; some problems may last for a short period of time, and others may last a lot longer. Mental health problems have a tendency to interfere with the normal development of a child or adolescent, and can affect their ability to function socially and/or psychologically.

Types

Disorders that occur specifically during childhood include:

- hyperkinetic disorders;
- conduct disorders;
- emotional disorders;
- social functioning disorders;
- pervasive development disorders (such as autism spectrum disorder, as defined in APA 2013);
- other disorders, such as enuresis or encopresis.

There are also mental disorders that can start in childhood; these include:

- depression;
- anxiety disorders;
- adjustment disorders;
- psychotic disorders;
- sleep problems.

Disorders that occur in adolescence include:

- conduct disorders;
- eating disorders;
- mood disorders;
- anxiety disorders;
- obsessive compulsive disorder;
- schizophrenia;
- substance misuse.

Self-harm is common in adolescence; it is reported that 1 in 12 adolescents self-harm, with overdosing on paracetamol the most common known method (Geddes *et al*. 2012 and http://www.mentalhealth.org.uk/help-information/mental-health-a-z/s/self-harm).

Clinical features

Mental health problems in children and adolescents can present in different ways according to age and on this basis it is important that a full assessment is carried out, which should include:

- interviewing the child or adolescent, their parents or carers, and their teachers;
- assessing their psychological, social and physical functioning and development;
- considering the family structure;
- assessment for signs of abuse or neglect.

Risk factors

The prevalence of mental health disorders in children and adolescents is 10–20 per cent in the UK (Katona *et al.* 2012), with a higher prevalence in boys than girls. Factors that increase an individual's risk include:

- a co-morbid genetic disorder;
- physical health problems;
- poor educational performance;
- a co-morbid mental health disorder;
- family difficulties;
- overprotective parents;
- parents with a mental health problem;
- stress or trauma;
- abuse or neglect;
- bullying;
- loss.

Management

The management of mental health problems in children and adolescents is dependent on the presentation and also the level of complexity. Child and adolescent mental health services in the UK are therefore designed around a tiered system.

- Tier 1 — interventions are provided by practitioners who are not mental health specialists and who work in universal services.
- Tier 2 — interventions are provided by mental health practitioners working in the community or primary-care teams.
- Tier 3 — interventions are provided by mental health teams for children and adolescents with severe, complex and persistent mental health needs.
- Tier 4 — interventions are provided as in Tier 3, but a higher level of risk has been identified.

  Treatment guidelines recommend:

- cognitive behavioural therapy;
- family therapy;
- group and individual therapy;
- solution-focused therapy.

Psychological interventions

When working with children and adolescents with mental health problems the mental health nurse might be supervised by a specialist in this area, or they may be required to follow an agreed plan of care which might include:

- engaging and supporting recovery therapeutically;
- taking a strengths approach;

- working in partnership;
- listening and respecting the individual's experiences.

Dementia

Definition

Dementia is a syndrome rather than a specific diagnosis and it is therefore important to recognise that there are different types of dementia with different causes and presentations. In *The Diagnostic and Statistical Manual of Mental Disorders*, Fifth Edition [APA 2013] dementia is now described as a major neurocognitive disorder. The dementias are organic disorders which result from an identified biological cause.

Types

The types of dementia include:

- Alzheimer's disease;
- vascular dementia;
- Parkinson's disease;
- dementia in Pick's disease;
- dementia in Creutzfeldt–Jakob disease;
- dementia in Huntington's disease;
- dementia in human immunodeficiency virus (HIV);
- post-encephalitic dementia;
- head-trauma-related dementia;
- alcohol-related dementia.

  Dementia is diagnosed when the following are observed:

- multiple cognitive impairments, including memory, orientation, language, comprehension and reasoning;
- a decline in social functioning;
- clear consciousness.

Clinical features

Dementia may present as a progressive decline in cognition and social functioning; however it may also have a sudden onset (or appear to). The clinical features of the dementias include:

- apathy;
- aggression;
- restlessness;
- disinhibition;
- impulsivity;
- low mood;
- anxiety;
- delusion;

- hallucinations;
- sleep disturbances.

Risk factors

Dementia becomes more prevalent with increasing age; the prevalence of dementia is less than 1% before the age of 65, increasing to 25% by the age of 90 (Geddes *et al.* 2012, Katona *et al.* 2012). Alzheimer's disease is the most common dementia, accounting for 55% of all dementias; vascular dementia accounts for about 25% (Geddes *et al.* 2012, Katona *et al.* 2012). In addition to age, other factors that increase an individual's risk include:

- genetics;
- family history;
- Down's syndrome;
- cardiovascular problems;
- an unhealthy diet;
- a lack of physical activity;
- smoking;
- high levels of alcohol consumption;
- social isolation;
- head injury.

Management

Early diagnosis and early intervention in dementia is important, especially when other mental disorders, such a depression, are also present. In terms of specific interventions treatment guidelines recommend:

- anti-dementia medication;
- cognitive stimulation;
- reality orientation therapy;
- validation therapy;
- behavioural therapy.

Psychological interventions

When nursing an individual diagnosed with a dementia it is important to consider that the environment has a significant role to play in keeping an individual well. Changes to an environment can compensate in part for reduced sensory, cognitive and motor ability. It is also important to ensure that an individual's physical needs are not neglected. The types of interventions the mental health nurse may deliver include:

- establishing a therapeutic relationship based on a person-centred approach;

- providing tailored support that focuses on assisting the individual to meet their physical needs;
- working on improving cognitive ability, including memory;
- reducing disorientation through memory prompts, both verbal and environmental;
- being empathetic to the emotional context and meaning of someone experiencing memory loss and confusion;
- provide behavioural strategies that positively modify challenging behaviour.

Depression

Definition
Depression is classed as a mood disorder in which low mood is a common symptom. This is not necessarily the same as normal sadness, which might occur after bereavement, a serious physical illness, or after a traumatic event.

Types
The diagnosis of depression is characterised by levels of severity.

- Mild — the symptoms are less intense (a clinical judgment), but still have some impact upon social functioning.
- Moderate — more symptoms are present and there is a greater impact upon social functioning.
- Severe — the individual has a persistent low mood and the symptoms are so distressing the individual finds it difficult to function.

Clinical features
An individual can have a single or a recurrent depressive episode; a recurrent episode is when an individual has experienced more than one depressive episode. When psychotic symptoms, such as hallucinations and delusions, are present depression is always described as severe. A diagnosis of depression is assigned if at least two of the three core symptoms are present every day for two weeks:

- low mood;
- loss of interest;
- low energy.

Associated symptoms can include:

- disturbed sleep;
- poor concentration;
- low self-confidence;
- poor appetite;
- suicidal thoughts or acts;

- agitation;
- slowing of movements;
- guilt.

The severity of the episode of depression depends on the:

- number of symptoms;
- severity of the symptoms and the degree of distress;
- impact upon social functioning.

Individuals can experience a range of cognitive, behavioural and physical symptoms. It is not uncommon for individuals to have negative thoughts about:

- themselves — low self-esteem;
- the world and others;
- their future.

They may also have thoughts that relate to death and suicide.

Risk factors

Depression is a common disorder and the estimated lifetime risk can range from 10 to 20 per cent. Prevalence is influenced by gender, age and marital status; depression is higher in women, older adults and individuals living in areas that are classed as deprived. A number of factors increase an individual's risk:

- family history of depression;
- psychosocial factors, such as loss of employment, parental loss, lack of a confiding relationship;
- severe physical illness;
- childbirth;
- a genetic predisposition.

Management

Depression is usually treated within a primary-care setting without the need to refer to psychiatric services unless the risk to self and/or others is high, the individual has severe depression that is unresponsive to treatment, or the depressive episode is recurrent or part of a bipolar presentation. In terms of interventions, current treatment guidelines recommend:

- cognitive behavioural therapy;
- interpersonal therapy;
- guided self-help;
- self-help groups;
- structured physical activity;
- behavioural activation;

- antidepressants;
- electroconvulsive therapy in severe cases.

Psychological interventions

A mental health nurse will work with individuals who have been diagnosed with mild, moderate or severe depression and it is therefore important that the nurse follows the stepped-care model, which is designed to indicate the choice of intervention by the severity of the depressive episode. Before the nurse delivers any specific psychological interventions they will need to ensure that they have built an effective therapeutic relationship; they will also need to manage any identified risk and/or any co-morbid conditions. The types of interventions the nurse might deliver include:

- cognitive restructuring;
- behavioural activation;
- problem-solving;
- relapse prevention;
- psychosocial interventions;
- motivational interviewing;
- guided self-help.

Disorders associated with pregnancy

Definition

Most women have good mental health during pregnancy. Some women may already have a mental illness when they get pregnant, and some will develop a mental illness during pregnancy; depression and anxiety are the most common mental health problems in pregnancy. However, more serious mental health conditions, such as bipolar affective disorder, severe depression and psychosis can occur during both pregnancy and the postnatal period. How the woman's mental health is affected during pregnancy depends on:

- the type of mental health problem previously experienced;
- whether a woman is currently undergoing treatment for a mental illness;
- recent stressful events in in a woman's life;
- how the woman feels about the pregnancy.

Types

The most common mental disorders in pregnancy include:

- anxiety;
- depression;
- psychosis;

Clinical features

Individuals with an anxiety disorder during pregnancy can experience a range of cognitive, behavioural and physical symptoms depending on the condition:

- fear and worry;
- increased vigilance;
- irritability and restlessness;
- poor concentration;
- sleeping difficulties;
- physical tension;
- hyperactivity;
- palpitations;
- abdominal discomfit and nausea;
- hot flushes;
- outbursts of anger;
- ruminating thoughts and compulsions.

Depression can occur at any stage during pregnancy and symptoms may include:

- low mood;
- loss of interest;
- low energy.

Associated symptoms include:

- disturbed sleep;
- poor concentration;
- low self-confidence;
- poor appetite;
- suicidal thoughts or acts;
- agitation;
- slowing of movements;
- guilt.

Postnatal depression is not clinically distinct from depression; the only difference is that the individual has recently given birth. Puerperal psychosis (also known as post-partum psychosis) is not recognised as a distinct disorder, but symptoms include delusions, hallucinations, disorganised thinking, grossly disorganised or abnormal motor behaviour, and negative symptoms (a loss of normal functions).

Risk factors

Prevalence rates of mental health problems during pregnancy are around 9% (Geddes *et al*. 2012, Katona *et al*. 2012); however, this figure might be underestimated due to low diagnostic rates. Risk is increased where the individual has:

- a pre-existing mental illness, such as schizophrenia, bipolar disorder, schizoaffective disorder or severe depression;
- had previous treatment from mental health services;
- a previous postpartum psychosis or severe postnatal depression;
- a severe anxiety disorder such as obsessive compulsive disorder;
- an eating disorder, such as anorexia or bulimia.

Management

Depression and anxiety can be treated as separate or co-morbid conditions and are generally managed effectively within primary care. More serious mental health conditions that occur during or after pregnancy might require input from secondary care services, such as assessment or admission to a specialist perinatal unit. The general practitioner, health visitor and midwife will, of course, play vital roles as part of a multidisciplinary approach. Psychotropic medication and psychological therapies (talking treatments) can help with anxiety, depression and more serious mental health conditions during pregnancy. Although there is national guidance on anxiety and depression, there are specific recommendations for pregnant women.

- Anxiety during pregnancy:
  - low-intensity psychological interventions, such as facilitated self-help;
  - high-intensity psychological interventions, such as cognitive behavioural therapy (CBT);
  - medications management;
  - in cases of tokophobia (extreme fear of childbirth) it is essential to involve the wider perinatal team.
- Depression during pregnancy:
  - antidepressant medication;
  - high-intensity psychological interventions, such as CBT.
- Serious mental illness during pregnancy:
  - CBT;
  - individual psychotherapy;
  - couples therapy (bipolar);
  - antipsychotic therapy;
  - family interventions (psychoses).

Psychological interventions

Mental health nurses work in a variety of clinical settings and will work with women who have been diagnosed with a mental health disorder during or after pregnancy. A key role of the mental health nurse is to work closely with universal services to ensure that risks are being assessed and monitored. Before the nurse can deliver any specific psychological interventions they will need to ensure that they have built an effective therapeutic relationship. Discussions and decisions around care should involve families and partners where possible. It is imperative that health professionals acknowledge the woman's role in caring for her baby during times of mental distress and offer support and compassion in a non-judgmental way.

Depending on the skill and training of the nurse the types of interventions the nurse might deliver are:

- supportive counselling;
- CBT;
- physical well-being (including weight, smoking, nutrition, activity, alcohol);
- relaxation therapy;
- psychoeducation on the topics of breastfeeding and psychotropic medication.

Drug misuse

Definition

Drug misuse occurs when an individual's drug use has a harmful impact, with the potential to cause physical, social and psychological harms. The individual may or may not be dependent on the drug/s; signs of dependency include:

- compulsion to take the drug;
- adverse impact upon the individual's social functioning;
- the individual becomes tolerant to the drug;
- the individual has difficulty controlling their drug use;
- the individual experiences withdrawal symptoms when stopping their drug use.

Illicit drugs can generally be divided into the following categories:

- opiates;
- stimulants;
- hallucinogens;
- cannabis.

Types

Drug disorders include:

- acute intoxication;
- harmful use;
- dependence;
- withdrawal state;
- psychotic disorder;
- amnesic disorder.

Clinical features

The clinical presentation of drug misuse depends on the type of drug; opiates can cause drowsiness whereas stimulants can cause restlessness. Generally, substance misuse can lead to:

- disturbed consciousness and perception;
- damage to an individual's health and social functioning;
- neglect;
- physical and psychological withdrawal;
- hallucinations and delusions;
- memory and cognitive impairments.

Risk factors

It is estimated that one in ten adults in the UK have used an illicit substance: cannabis is the most commonly used drug. The causes of drug misuse are not clear, but there are factors that increase an individual's risk:

- availability of the substance;
- peer pressure;
- a co-morbid mental health disorder;
- stressful situations or circumstances;
- family history;
- life events, such as childhood abuse and loss.

Management

The management of substance misuse is dependent on the presentation and the drug/s being used; an individual can present with signs of acute intoxication, withdrawal or dependency. In terms of specific interventions current treatment guidelines recommend:

- acute detoxification;
- motivational enhancement therapy;
- cognitive behavioural therapy;
- abstinence;
- social learning strategies;
- harm-reduction strategies;
- self-help groups;
- medication to manage cravings.

Psychological interventions

It is important to note that an individual's substance use can change over time, and they may spontaneously stop their drug misuse. Service users who misuse drugs are usually treated outside of the mental health inpatient setting; however, mental health nurses will encounter individuals who both misuse drugs and have a co-morbid mental health disorder. After the detoxification phase the mental health nurse will need to deliver different types of psychological interventions, which include:

- building a collaborative and therapeutic relationship;
- motivational and brief intervention work;
- guided self-help;
- harm reduction;
- coping strategy work;
- health promotion;
- family and couples work;
- contingency approaches — using incentives to change behaviour.

Eating disorders

Definition
The term "eating disorder" indicates that an individual has abnormal eating habits, which can range from not eating enough food to eating food in excess. These abnormal eating habits impact adversely on the individual's health and well-being.

Types
The most common eating disorders are:

- anorexia nervosa — a morbid fear of fatness;
- bulimia nervosa — morbid fear of fatness with binge eating;
- binge-eating disorder — binge eating without purging.

   An eating disorder diagnosis is usually assigned if the individual conforms to the following descriptions.

- Anorexia nervosa — the individual has a morbid fear of fatness with a distorted body image, is deliberately losing weight (with a body mass index [BMI] less than 17.5) and has amenorrhoea.
- Bulimia nervosa — the individual has a morbid fear of fatness and a preoccupation with body weight, is binge eating on large amounts of food and is trying to prevent weight gain through such behaviours as vomiting and misusing laxatives.
- Binge-eating disorder — the individual is binge eating without purging and this behaviour is leading to obesity (measured by a BMI of 30 or above).

Clinical features
Eating disorders, especially anorexia nervosa and bulimia nervosa, are characterised by a preoccupation with weight and body image. Purging and binge eating can be present in anorexia nervosa; other features of anorexia nervosa include:

- being self-conscious about eating in public;
- dieting;
- excessive exercise;
- constipation;
- emaciation;
- dry skin;
- amenorrhoea;
- bradycardia and hypotension.

The clinical features of bulimia nervosa include:

- a craving for food;
- fluctuating weight;
- fasting;
- excessive exercise;
- intense loathing, especially after bingeing;
- amenorrhoea;
- acute oesophageal tears, which are related to vomiting.

Risk factors

Eating disorders primarily affect women; anorexia nervosa and bulimia nervosa are three times more common in women than in men. The prevalence rates for eating disorders range from 10 to 20 per cent of the population, and between one and three percent have a specific diagnosis. Risk factors that increase the risk of an individual developing the condition include:

- presence of an eating disorder amongst first-degree relatives;
- a first-degree relative who has an anxiety disorder, depression or an obsessional personality, or, in the case of bulimia nervosa, has a diagnosis of substance misuse;
- age — early adolescence is a risk factor for anorexia nervosa; the late teens have an increased risk for bulimia nervosa;
- low self esteem;
- difficulty in expressing emotions(this is specific to anorexia nervosa);
- being impulsive (this is specific to bulimia nervosa);
- having an upbringing where weight and food are overvalued;
- being bullied about their weight;
- experiencing life events such as childhood abuse and loss.

Management

The first-line treatment for adolescents with anorexia nervosa is family therapy, and for adults a number of therapies can be offered, including:

- cognitive behavioural therapy (CBT);
- interpersonal therapy;

- psychodynamic therapy;
- family therapy;
- medication — when depression is co-morbid with other mental health problems.

The first-line treatment for bulimia nervosa is usually CBT or interpersonal therapy; antidepressants can also be prescribed when depression is co-morbid with other mental health problems. Treatment for binge-eating disorder usually consists of CBT, exercise and nutritional education.

Psychological interventions

Individuals diagnosed with an eating disorder are usually treated outside of the inpatient setting. In the case of anorexia nervosa treatment within an inpatient setting might be required if there is a significant risk to self; this can be due to suicidal thoughts or the physical impact of the disorder. The mental health nurse might need to stabilise the individual's physical condition before instigating the following psychological interventions:

- building a collaborative and therapeutic relationship;
- motivational work;
- psychoeducation and guided self-help;
- behavioural work – specifically targeting weight gain;
- coping strategy work;
- family work.

Functional disorders in older adults

Definition

The UK has an increasingly aging population. Mental health services have historically been segregated into services for individuals under the age of 65 and services for individuals over the age of 65; however this artificial division is now changing to focus on providing services that are led by needs. In terms of functional disorders older adults have similar needs to younger adults and so they should be given a similar level of care. In general, a functional disorder is different to an organic disorder; organic disorders result from an identified biological cause whereas functional disorders have no apparent biological cause.

Types

Functional disorders in older adults include:

- personality disorders;
- depression;

- anxiety disorders;
- mania;
- psychotic disorders.

The assessment, diagnosis and management of these functional disorders is the same for older adults as for younger adults.

Clinical features

The normal aging process usually means that an individual experiences a number of changes that can be physical, psychological, social and spiritual. These changes, together with how society views the aging process, can have an impact upon the presentation, diagnosis and treatment of a given functional disorder:

- older adults are less likely to report low mood or suicidal thoughts;
- depression tends to be viewed as part of the aging process and, as a result, the appropriate treatment is not always given;
- certain psychiatric medications should be used with caution if there is a co-existing physical illness;
- traumatic events, such as a fall, or a physical illness, such as a stroke, can lead to the onset of a functional disorder;
- mania is more likely to present in terms of irritability rather than overt elation;
- older adults are at a higher risk of completed suicide than younger adults.

Risk factors

Depression and anxiety disorders are the most common functional disorders diagnosed in older adults; the prevalence of all the functional disorders, except bipolar disorder, increases with age. Similar to functional disorders in younger adults there are a number of factors that increase an older adult's risk of functional disorders:

- the presence of a dementia increases the risk of depression;
- physical illness increases the risk of depression or mania;
- being socially isolated increases the risk of depression or a psychotic disorder;
- being in a nursing home or residential care increases the risk of depression;
- being a carer for someone with dementia increases the risk of depression;
- traumatic events increase the risk of an anxiety disorder;
- loss can increase the risk of depression or a psychotic disorder.

Management

Treatment is dependent on the functional disorder and its presentation, the individual's circumstances and their specific needs. Ensuring the individual is not socially isolated is a key part of the recovery process. In terms of interventions, current treatment guidelines recommend:

- cognitive behavioural therapy — individual or group therapy;
- treating any underlying physical illnesses;
- guided self-help;
- psychoeducation;
- group therapy;
- structured physical activity;
- behavioural activation;
- relaxation techniques;
- psychiatric medication;
- electroconvulsive therapy in severe cases of depression.

Psychological interventions

When nursing an older adult diagnosed with a functional disorder it is important that the individual is thoroughly assessed. This includes establishing whether there is an underlying physical condition. In addition, the risk assessment and management process needs to be sensitive to the increased risk of completed suicide in older adults. Depending on the skill of the nurse the types of interventions that might be delivered are:

- establishing a collaborative therapeutic relationship;
- normalising an individual's experiences of mental distress;
- reducing distress by modifying thought processes and enhancing coping strategies;
- preventing social isolation and promoting social functioning;
- problem-solving;
- signposting to self-help and relevant support groups.

Learning disabilities in mental health

Definition

Learning disabilities, sometimes known as intellectual disabilities and formerly classified as mental retardation, can be described as a reduced intellectual ability that has an onset before adulthood and can adversely affect an individual's social functioning. A learning disability is classed as:

- profound — intelligence quotient (IQ) below 20;
- severe — IQ 20–34;
- moderate — IQ 35–49;
- mild — IQ 50–69;

Types

The majority of individuals with a learning disability do not have a co-morbid mental health disorder, but there is an increased likelihood of being diagnosed with the following disorders:

- depression;
- obsessive compulsive disorder;
- a phobia;
- schizophrenia;
- mania.

Diagnosing specific mental health disorders can be difficult if an individual has profound communication difficulties or when symptoms that would usually be attributed to an underlying mental health disorder are instead viewed as learning disability behaviours.

Clinical features

Individuals with a learning disability and a co-morbid mental health disorder are usually described as having a dual diagnosis. One problem with the use of this term is that it is vague but the term dual diagnosis can also refer to any individual who has more than one diagnosis, whether it be a mental health, learning disability or physical condition. Individuals with a dual diagnosis can experience a range of cognitive, behavioural and physical symptoms that include:

- self-harm;
- aggression;
- inappropriate sexual behaviour;
- disturbed sleep;
- restlessness;
- compulsions;
- tearfulness;
- hallucinations;
- paranoid delusions.

Risk factors

The prevalence of individuals with a learning disability is approximately 1.5% of the general population in the UK (Rea and Ridley 2012). Among individuals with a learning disability there is an increased prevalence of mental health problems, which ranges from 20–40%. There are a number of factors that increase the risk of an individual with a learning disability developing a mental health problem:

- unemployment;
- discrimination;

- abuse;
- poverty;
- drug and alcohol problems;
- sensory impairments.

Management

Treating individuals with both a learning disability and a mental health disorder is similar to the treatment delivered to an individual without a learning disability. Dependent on the presenting issues, specific treatments might include:

- behavioural approaches;
- cognitive behavioural therapy;
- antidepressants;
- interpersonal therapy;
- psychodynamic therapy;
- relaxation techniques;
- psychoeducation;
- art therapy;
- antipsychotic medication.

Psychological interventions

Individuals with a learning disability might have an existing package of support in place prior to being diagnosed with a co-morbid mental health disorder. If this is the case the mental health nurse needs to tailor any subsequent psychological interventions to complement the existing care package. This might mean that the mental health nurse has to work across agencies and different settings, both to deliver care directly, and to support and advise others who are delivering care. The types of psychological interventions the nurse might deliver include:

- building a collaborative and therapeutic relationship;
- managing risk;
- promoting social functioning;
- cognitive restructuring;
- behavioural activation;
- problem-solving;
- relapse prevention;
- breathing and relaxation exercises.

Neuropsychiatry

Definition

Neuropsychiatry is a subspeciality of psychiatry that involves both neurology and psychiatry and deals with mental disorders attributable to diseases of the nervous system; organic disorders.

Types

Focal neurological disorders include:

- brain injury and stroke;
- post-concussion syndrome;
- epilepsy;
- tumour.

    Autoimmune and inflammatory disorders include:

- multiple sclerosis (MS);
- disorders of the basal ganglia;
- sleep disorders;
- tic disorders.

    Infectious causes of neuropsychiatric symptoms include human immunodeficiency virus.

Clinical features

An organic disorder can often present the same clinical picture as a functional disorder. Symptoms may include changes to personality and behaviour, cognitive impairment and/or confusional states, changes to mood and psychoses. The symptomology will often be determined by the site of the brain that is involved and the duration of the illness. It is not uncommon for a person with a focal neurological disorder (particularly epilepsy) to experience some mental health issues, such as depression, anxiety, delirium and psychosis. Furthermore, there is an increased risk of suicide with a number of neuropsychiatric conditions.

Risk factors

Prevalence of neuropsychiatric disorders is hard to estimate because of the way in which mental disorders are classified. In some countries the dementias and childhood disorders are included within estimates. The prevalence of mental health problems in individuals with neurological problems or those who have sustained a head injury is estimated to be 20–50% (Geddes *et al.* 2012, Katona *et al.* 2012). Factors that increase the risk of experiencing a neuropsychiatric problem include:

- stroke;
- traumatic brain injury;
- tumours;
- alcohol and/or substance abuse;
- genetic factors (MS, Huntington's disease, Wilson's disease, Tourette's syndrome);
- depression;
- infection.

Management

In the first instance, an accurate and timely diagnosis is imperative. The main goal of treatment, however, is symptom control and the promotion of well-being. Treatment is dependent on both the presenting problem and the underlying neurological condition.

Psychological interventions

Due to the extent of neuropsychiatric conditions, mental health nurses are likely to find themselves working in a range of clinical specialities. The types of psychological interventions that can be delivered will vary depending on the skill of the nurse. In all circumstances, however, the nurse will focus on the development of a person-centred therapeutic relationship and, depending on the condition, will:

- promote the individual's capacity to maintain independence;
- deliver specific therapeutic approaches;
- offer psychoeducation for patients and their families;
- offer cognitive behavioural therapy;
- use dialectic behaviour therapy.

Personality disorders

Definition

The definition of normal and abnormal personalities is measured in terms of personality traits and specifically in terms of how an individual is or is not functioning in relation to these traits. Personality disorders can be defined as behaviour patterns that are enduring and deeply ingrained, deviating distinctly from what is culturally expected and leading to distress to self and/or others. Personality disorders are categorised using two different methods — using either three main clusters or nine types. Both methods of categorisation are similar, though some names are slightly different, and narcissistic personality disorder is not included in the type classification.

Types

The three main clusters and nine types (where no alternative name is given for the type, it has the same name as the cluster categorisation) are:

- cluster A — paranoid, schizoid and schizotypal;
- cluster B — antisocial (type: dissocial), borderline (type: emotionally unstable), histrionic and narcissistic (not included in types);
- cluster C — avoidant (type: anxious), dependant and obsessive compulsive (type: anankastic).

A personality disorder is diagnosed not only in terms of whether specific traits are present but also in terms of how severe these traits are, whether there is significant risk to self and/or others, and how the traits impact upon the individual's social functioning. There may be other reasons why a person is exhibiting a disordered personality, these include:

- personality changes due to a physical condition;
- personality changes due to a long-standing mental disorder, such a schizophrenia.

Clinical features

It is not uncommon for an individual to exhibit traits that can fall into more than one personality disorder cluster and/or type. It is also not uncommon for a personality disorder to be either co-morbid with another mental health disorder or to be misdiagnosed. On this basis it is important that a full and comprehensive assessment is undertaken and that any co-morbid disorders are also identified and treated. The following is a list of some of the personality traits that an individual diagnosed with a specific personality disorder can exhibit:

- paranoid — suspicious and excessively sensitive;
- schizoid — emotional coldness, little interest in other people;
- schizotypal — odd beliefs and unusual appearance;
- borderline — instability of mood, impulsive;
- histrionic — excessive attention seeking;
- narcissistic — grandiose and arrogant;
- antisocial — disregard of self and others;
- avoidant — feelings of inadequacy;
- dependent — submissive behaviour;
- obsessive compulsive — a preoccupation with orderliness.

Risk factors

The prevalence of personality disorders can range from 2 to 13%; some studies use an average of 5% for the general population in the UK; the prevalence is significantly higher in individuals being treated for a mental health disorder (Geddes *et al.* 2012, Katona *et al.* 2012). The factors that increase the risk of an individual developing a personality disorder include:

- problems in early childhood — abuse, neglect and trauma;
- family history, including similar personality traits within the family;
- presence of other mental health problems;
- lack of adequate support for childhood traumas;
- unhealthy coping strategies.

Management

The management of individuals with a personality disorder has, in the past, been influenced by concerns over the success of treatment. There are now a number of interventions that show promise in the treatment of individuals diagnosed with a personality disorder, especially when the diagnosis is either a borderline or an antisocial personality disorder. These treatments include:

- cognitive behavioural therapy – group and individual therapy;
- behavioural approaches;
- mentalisation-based approaches;
- dialectic behaviour therapy;
- therapeutic community treatments.

Psychological interventions

Mental health nurses working with individuals diagnosed with a personality disorder need to consider risk, especially suicide. When the individual is a risk to self and/or others the mental health nurse will first implement psychological interventions that manage the identified risk; this could include the use of medication. At the same time the mental health nurse will work with the individual to build a therapeutic relationship. In the long term this relationship will be a vehicle for specific therapeutic approaches that assist the individual to regulate their own behaviour. Depending on the skill of the nurse the types of psychological interventions that can be delivered include:

- interventions that maintain safety and manage challenging behaviours effectively — boundary setting;
- focusing on the individual controlling and regulating their behaviour — promoting healthy ways of coping;
- exploring the individual's capacity to change — motivational interviewing and pre-therapy work;
- delivering specific therapeutic approaches/therapies.

Schizophrenia

Definition

Schizophrenia as a medical label originates from the work of Kraepelin in 1893, who coined the term 'dementia praecox' believing that schizophrenia was an early form of dementia (Carney and Smith 2012). In 1911, Bleuler, building on the work of Kraepelin but moving away from the idea of schizophrenia being an early form of dementia, first used the term schizophrenia; 'schiz' meaning 'split' and 'phren' meaning 'mind' (Carney and Smith 2012). Schizophrenia is medically classified as a psychotic disorder, the psychotic disorders also include:

- schizoaffective disorder;
- delusional disorder;
- brief psychotic episodes;
- psychotic depression;
- bipolar affective disorder;
- drug-induced psychosis.

Types
Schizophrenia is usually divided into subtypes, however this is not the case in *The Diagnostic and Statistical Manual of Mental Disorders*, Fifth Edition (APA 2013), which does not use these subtypes:

- disorganised (previously known as hebephrenic);
- catatonic;
- paranoid;
- residual;
- undifferentiated.

A diagnosis of schizophrenia is assigned if at least two of the following symptoms are present for a significant portion of time within a one-month period:

- hallucinations;
- delusions;
- disorganised speech;
- catatonic behaviour;
- disorganised behaviour;
- negative symptoms.

Clinical features
In terms of symptoms there are positive symptoms, which are distortions of normal functioning:

- hallucinations;
- delusions;
- thought disorders.

There are also negative symptoms, which involve the loss of normal functioning:

- lack of volition;
- poverty of thought and/or speech.

Both positive and negative symptoms can adversely impact greatly upon an individual's personal, social and occupational functioning.

The symptoms can also be experienced over a long period of time with frequent relapses even when antipsychotic medication is being taken.

Risk factors

Approximately 1% of the population in the UK have a diagnosis of schizophrenia (Geddes *et al*. 2012, Katona *et al*. 2012). The causes of schizophrenia are not clear, but there are a number of factors that increase the risk of an individual developing the condition:

- incidence of schizophrenia amongst first-degree relatives;
- age — there is a higher prevalence between the ages of 16 and 40;
- gender – early onset is more common in men;
- poor prenatal nutrition;
- obstetric complications;
- low social class;
- substance misuse — particularly stimulants.

Management

Early detection and early intervention are important in the diagnosis and successful treatment of schizophrenia, especially in the case of a first episode if an individual presents with a very acute and sudden onset. In terms of interventions, current treatment guidelines recommend:

- cognitive behavioural therapy;
- family interventions;
- art therapy;
- support groups;
- antipsychotic medication.

Psychological interventions

When nursing an individual with a diagnosis of schizophrenia a mental health nurse needs to be able to deliver a range of psychological interventions. When there is an increased risk of harm to others and/or to self, including self-neglect, the nurse should also develop appropriate risk-management strategies. This does not mean that risky behaviour is an inherent part of the diagnosis of schizophrenia. It may be the case that, in the short term, the individual is high risk to self because they are experiencing uncontrolled psychotic symptoms and struggling to keep themselves safe. In the long term, increased risk is more likely to be related physical health factors, such as poor diet, little exercise, obesity and smoking, leading to an increased risk of mortality. While managing risk the nurse should start to deliver psychological interventions that are shaped by a cognitive behavioural approach:

- establish a collaborative and therapeutic relationship;
- normalise psychotic experiences;
- reduce psychotic symptoms by modifying thought processes and enhancing coping strategies;
- prevent social isolation;
- promote social functioning;
- focus on relapse prevention;
- alleviate symptoms.

Sexual disorders

Definition
Sexual disorder is the impairment of normal sexual functioning. This can be the inability to reach orgasm, painful intercourse, repulsion to sexual activity or an exaggerated sexual response cycle or sexual interest. A medical cause must be excluded prior to making any sexual dysfunction diagnosis and the symptoms must be such that an individual's day-to-day functioning is impaired.

Types
Sexual disorders can be categorised as follows:

- erectile dysfunction (ED);
- premature ejaculation;
- delayed ejaculation (male orgasmic disorder);
- retrograde ejaculation;
- female orgasmic disorder;
- vaginismus;
- female sexual arousal disorder;
- dyspareunia;
- hypoactive sexual desire disorder (HSDD);
- gender identity disorder.

Clinical features
Clinical features of sexual disorders are outlined below.

- ED is often referred to as impotence and is the inability to achieve and maintain an erection. ED is a common condition amongst older men and estimates suggest that over half of all men between the ages of 40 and 70 will have it to some degree (http://www.nhs.uk/livewell/goodsex/pages/malesexualdysfunction.aspx).
- Premature ejaculation is the most common ejaculation problem and occurs when the man ejaculates too quickly during intercourse.

The condition can cause frustration and shame, and can impact on relationships, sexual intimacy and quality of life.

- Delayed ejaculation can be classified as experiencing a significant delay before ejaculation is possible or being unable to ejaculate at all (even though the man may want to and his erection is normal).
- Retrograde ejaculation is a rarer form of ejaculatory problem; it happens when the sperm travels backwards and enters the bladder. The main symptoms are producing no semen and producing cloudy urine. The condition does not pose any danger to health and men can still experience orgasm; however, it can effect fertility.
- Female orgasmic disorder is when a woman either cannot reach orgasm or has trouble reaching orgasm when she is sexually excited.
- Vaginismus is the term used to describe persistent or recurrent involuntary tightening of the muscles around the vagina whenever penetration is attempted. The condition can also make gynaecological examination extremely difficult.
- Female sexual arousal disorder describes a lack of sexual response to sexual stimulation.
- Dyspareunia is painful sexual intercourse, due to either medical or psychological reasons.
- HSDD is characterised by a lack of sexual desire (libido) and no interest in sexual activity. It effects both men and women.
- Gender identity disorder has also been placed in this category, although no outward dysfunction needs to be present for this disorder. Gender identity disorder describes strong feelings of being the wrong gender, or feelings that the outward body is inconsistent with the internal sense of being either male or female.

Risk factors

Naturally, the risk factors for sexual disorders vary according to the specific condition and whether it applies to a man or a woman:

- prostate problems;
- type 2 diabetes;
- hypertension;
- vascular disease;
- high levels of cholesterol;
- alcohol and substance misuse;
- smoking;

- advancing age;
- depression;
- infection;
- medications (e.g. antipsychotics);
- obesity;
- stress;

Management
In the first instance, the management of sexual disorders should treat any underlying organic or psychological cause. In the second instance, the management goal is for the individual to have a fulfilling sexual life.

Psychological interventions
Mental health nurses may be asked to support an individual experiencing a sexual disorder. Many antipsychotic medications can cause sexual side effects such as ED, and depression can often include sexual symptoms such as loss of libido. A person-centred therapeutic relationship will make conversations easier for what some may consider to being an embarrassing or sensitive topic. It is most likely that the nurse will signpost the person to the most appropriate service, but a basic knowledge of the treatment options is useful:

- ED medication;
- healthy lifestyles (regular exercise, quitting smoking and modifying alcohol intake);
- couples counselling;
- psychosexual counselling;
- cognitive behavioural therapy;
- lubrication;
- changes in sexual position (to alleviate discomfort or enhance pleasure);
- vacuum pumps;
- penile implants;
- pelvic floor exercises;
- complementary therapies.

Sleep disorders

Definition
Sleep disorders are problems associated with sleeping, including difficulty in falling asleep, staying asleep, falling asleep at the wrong time, sleeping too much or experiencing abnormal behaviours

during sleep. Persistent sleep disorders can often lead to poor mental health, such as anxiety and depression, and in extreme cases psychosis.

Types
Sleep disorders include:

- problems falling and staying asleep (insomnia);
- problems staying awake (hypersomnia);
- problems sticking to a regular sleep schedule (irregular sleep–wake syndrome, jet-lag syndrome, paradoxical insomnia, shift-work sleep disorder);
- unusual behaviours during sleep (parasomnias).

Clinical features
Clinical features of sleep disorders are dependent on the presenting problem.

- Insomnia — trouble falling asleep or staying asleep. Often the person wakes up early, feels tired and irritable and unable to cope or function during the day. Episodes may come and go and can be short or long lasting. Insomnia can be categorised according to duration:
  - short-term insomnia lasts less than four weeks;
  - long-term (persistent) insomnia last for four weeks or longer.
- Hypersomnia — excessive sleep or sleepiness during that day that interferes with day-to-day functioning. There are many possible reasons for this; sleep apnoea (interruption of normal breathing during sleep), restless leg syndrome, severe sleep deprivation, some medications, drug and alcohol misuse or previous head injury.
- Irregular sleep–wake syndrome — this disorder is extremely rare and involves sleeping or napping during the day, trouble falling asleep at night and often waking up in the night. It usually occurs in in people who do not have a regular routine during the day. The amount of sleep is usually normal, but the body clock loses its normal circadian cycle. Shift workers and travellers who change time zones are most effected.
- Parasomnias — a cluster of sleep disorders that involve unwanted events or experiences that occur while falling asleep, during sleep or on waking up. Parasomnias include abnormal movements, sleep walking, sleep talking, sleep terrors, bedwetting and rapid eye

movement sleep disturbance, such as acting-out dreams. A person who experiences parasomnia often has no recollection of the events that took place during sleep.

Risk factors

The prevalence of sleep disorders is difficult to measure as they are not always reported; however, it is estimated that 20–50% of adults report sleeping difficulties with a higher prevalence in women and older adults (https://sleepfoundation.org/sleepdisorders-problems). Risk factors for sleep disorders include:

- increasing age;
- lifestyle;
- environment;
- diet (including caffeine intake);
- drugs and alcohol;
- stress and worry;
- anxiety and depression;
- psychological trauma;
- mental illness;
- hormonal changes (women);
- obesity;
- physical illness and pain;
- some prescription medications.

Management

The priority for the management of sleep disorders should be to first identify and treat any identifiable underlying cause. A detailed sleep assessment can provide a baseline and this can take place in the home or care environment. Dedicated sleep centres can offer electronic monitoring of sleep. Medication and talking therapies can be offered independently or in combination as an effective solution to many sleep disorders.

Psychological interventions

It is important to remember that, although anyone can experience sleep disorder at some point in their lives, mental illness and sleep disturbance share a symbiotic relationship with one another. Whether a person cannot sleep because of their psychological distress or whether they have become mentally distressed on account of being unable to sleep does not matter. The goal of treatment is to address the sleep disturbance and any underlying psychological issues. Mental health nurses and practitioners are well placed to offer psychoeducation and helpful interventions to promote sleep:

- sleep hygiene:
  - establish fixed times for going to bed and waking up;
  - engage in relaxation before bedtime;
  - ensure bedroom is comfortable; not too hot/cold/draughty/noisy;
  - avoid napping during the day;
  - avoid caffeine, nicotine and alcohol before going to bed;
  - avoid exercise for four hours before going to bed;
  - avoid eating meals late at night;
  - only use the bedroom for sleep or sexual activity.
- stimulation-control therapy;
- paradoxical intention;
- biofeedback;
- relaxation therapy;
- sleep-restriction therapy;
- lifestyle changes;
- hypnotic medication, antidepressant medication, melatonin;
- complementary therapies (including acupuncture and herbal remedies).

Trauma and other stress-related conditions

Definition
Unlike other disorders, trauma and other stress-related conditions have a causative element. Stress-related conditions include reactive attachment disorder, disinhibited social engagement disorder, post-traumatic stress disorder (PTSD), acute stress disorder and adjustment disorder.

Types
Trauma and other stress-related conditions can be categorised into five types.

- Reactive attachment disorder (only present in children) — a child withdraws emotionally from social contact due to abuse, neglect etc.
- Disinhibited social engagement disorder — a child becomes unreserved in their interactions with unfamiliar adults due to abuse, neglect etc.
- PTSD — a fearful response to a threatening and/or catastrophic event, which is re-experienced through upsetting thoughts or memories and leads to avoiding certain situations; the individual

may have difficulty sleeping, feel irritable and have difficulty concentrating (the symptoms must have lasted for more than a month).

- Acute stress disorder — similar to PTSD, but symptoms must be experienced for more than three days and less than one month. If symptoms last more than one month then a diagnosis of PTSD is applied.
- Adjustment disorder — a stressor, such as distress at work and/or home, leads to anxiety and/or depression longer than is expected for most people. The disorder starts within three months of the stressor starting and stops within six months of the stressor ending.

Clinical features

Individuals with stress-related conditions can experience a range of cognitive, behavioural and physical symptoms, depending on the condition, including:

- fear and worry;
- increased vigilance;
- irritability and restlessness;
- poor concentration;
- sleeping difficulties;
- physical tension;
- hyperactivity;
- palpitations;
- abdominal discomfort and nausea;
- hot flushes;
- outbursts of anger;
- low mood.

Risk factors

The prevalence of stress-related conditions where there has been a trauma are as high as 70% with an average of 40% in the general population (NICE 2011). There are a number of factors that increase an individual's risk of stress-related conditions, including:

- substance misuse;
- social isolation;
- life events, such as childhood abuse, loss of employment, parental loss, excessive demands or high expectations, or witnessing traumatic event.

Management

The treatment of stress-related disorders, similar to the treatment of anxiety disorders, usually occurs within a primary-care setting. Specific interventions are dependent on the condition and the individual's preference. Current treatment guidelines recommend:

- cognitive behavioural therapy (CBT) including trauma-focused CBT;
- behavioural therapy;
- medication, such as selective serotonin re-uptake inhibitors;
- interpersonal therapy;
- group therapy;
- psychodynamic therapy;
- mindfulness approaches;
- systemic therapy;
- eye movement desensitisation;
- relaxation techniques.

Psychological interventions

Mental health nurses work in a variety of settings and they will encounter individuals who have been diagnosed with a stress-related disorder both as a disorder on its own and as a co-morbid disorder. It is not uncommon for a stress-related disorder to be co-morbid with other disorders, such as depression, substance misuse or an anxiety disorder. Risk needs to be managed as part of the delivery of any psychological intervention as well as ensuring that an effective therapeutic relationship has been built. Depending on the skill and training of the nurse the types of interventions that can be delivered are:

- guided self-help;
- breathing and relaxation exercises;
- identifying, challenging and replacing negative thoughts;
- motivational interviewing;
- desensitisation.

Unresolved grief

Definition

Bereavement is a distressing but common experience; we grieve after loss. After the death of a loved one people can experience;

- being stunned;
- emotional numbness;
- anger;
- guilt;
- agitation.

Most people recover from a major bereavement within one or two years, but some people experience unresolved grief. This can be the case when their grief is;

- prolonged beyond six months;
- delayed in onset;
- more intense than you would normally expect to see.

It is not unusual for a person to present with depression and, on assessment, the depression is linked to a recent loss.

Types
Types of unresolved grief include:

- unresolved or complicated grief;
- anticipatory and disenfranchised grief.

Clinical features
Although many of the symptoms identified as unresolved grief can be considered ordinary during the more acute earlier phase of grief, they are considered major signs of unresolved/complicated grief if they remain for unusually prolonged periods of time. After the death of someone close a number of the following symptoms are present:

- persistent yearning for the deceased;
- intense sorrow and emotional pain in response to the death;
- preoccupation with the deceased;
- preoccupation with the circumstances of the death;
- marked difficulty accepting the death;
- disbelief or emotional numbness over the loss;
- difficulty reminiscing positively about the deceased;
- bitterness or anger related to the loss;
- maladaptive appraisals about oneself in relation to the deceased or the death (e.g. self-blame);
- excessive avoidance of reminders of the loss;
- a desire to die to be with the deceased;
- difficulty trusting other people since the death;
- feeling alone or detached from other people since the death;
- feeling that life is meaningless or empty without the deceased or the belief that one cannot function without the deceased;
- confusion about one's role in life or a diminished sense of one's identity;
- difficulty or reluctance to pursue interests or to plan for the future (e.g. friendships, activities) since the loss.

In addition, the disturbance causes clinically significant distress or impairment in social, occupational, or other important areas of functioning, and the bereavement reaction must be out of proportion or inconsistent with cultural or religious norms.

Risk factors

The prevalence of unresolved grief within the bereaved population is reported to be around 15% (Guldin *et al*. 2013); it is greater if there has been a major disaster, and it is more likely to occur with the loss of a child or where violence has been a factor. There are a number of factors that increase an individual's risk of experiencing unresolved grief:

* a history of mental health problems;
* a family history of mental health problems;
* a history of substance misuse;
* death of child;
* death of a partner;
* cot death;
* unexpected death;
* traumatic death;
* social isolation.

Management

Unresolved grief is usually treated within a primary-care setting. In terms of specific interventions there is no evidence that one approach is more effective than another; however, an individual might have a co-morbid mental health condition that would also need treating. The following interventions might be appropriate:

* bereavement counselling;
* cognitive behavioural therapy for traumatic grief;
* brief psychotherapy;
* internet-based interventions;
* self-help guides and groups;
* medication — short-term use for sleep problems.

Psychological interventions

Mental health nurses will encounter individuals who have been diagnosed with unresolved grief; most will have a co-morbid disorder such as depression and/or post-traumatic stress. Risk needs to be managed as part of the delivery of any psychological intervention as well as ensuring that an effective therapeutic relationship has been built. Depending on the skill and training of the nurse, the types of interventions that can be delivered are:

- guided self-help;
- breathing and relaxation exercises;
- identifying, challenging and replacing negative thoughts;
- cognitive restructuring;
- behavioural activation;
- problem-solving;
- psychosocial interventions.

Specific issues

Rapid Mental Health Nursing, First Edition. Grahame Smith and Rebecca Rylance.
© 2016 John Wiley & Sons, Ltd. Published 2016 by John Wiley & Sons, Ltd.

Asylum seekers and refugees

Background

An asylum seeker is a person who flees their homeland and arrives at another country by any way they can. Upon arrival they make themselves known to the authorities and lodge an application for refugee protection on the basis of the *Refugee Convention 1951* or Article 3 of the *European Convention on Human Rights 2010*, which states that, 'No one shall be subjected to torture or inhuman or degrading treatment or punishment'.

According to Article 3 of the *European Convention on Human Rights 2010*, member states are prohibited from returning a person to a country where he/she may suffer a violation of his/her rights under Article 3. In the UK, an asylum seeker can legally stay in the country while the authorities determine whether they can stay or not. A refugee has had their claim for protection approved by the government and can stay in the country long term or indefinitely. This is known as 'leave to remain'. Anyone waiting for a decision is entitled to free primary and secondary care health services. It is recognised that the process of fleeing from a homeland and waiting for confirmation of 'leave to remain' is incredibly stressful and traumatic. Often, asylum seekers have fled their countries following torture and fearful situations, and many asylum seekers experience post-traumatic stress disorder.

Implications for practice

In addition to numerous social complexities, such as poor housing and employment, language barriers, poor social engagement and isolation, racism and family separation, many asylum seekers and refugees experience significant mental health issues. The conditions listed below are thought to be prevalent, according to a report by Mind (2009):

- HIV–AIDS;
- postnatal depression;
- substance misuse;
- female genital mutilation;
- anxiety and depression.

The challenge when caring for asylum seekers and refugees with mental health issues is that their understanding and interpretation of mental health may be quite different to the beliefs held in the UK, and may not necessarily fit with their needs. Furthermore, cultural and religious taboos can be a barrier and therefore affect their engagement with mental health services (Mind 2009); and of course this may be compounded by stigma and fear.

The role of the mental health nurse

The role of mental health nurse when working with asylum seekers and refugees includes:

- working with refugee community organisations;
- establishing links between refugees and established cultural groups, such as church or social groups;
- educating and signposting the refugee to appropriate mental health services;
- challenging stigma and encouraging refugees to access primary-care services.

Culture and ethnicity

Background

Different ethnic groups have different experiences and rates of mental health issues, reflecting their different cultural and social economic contexts (http://www.mentalhealth.org.uk/help-information/mental-health-a-z/B/BME-communities/). Generally speaking, in the UK black and minority ethnic (BME) groups are more likely to be diagnosed with a mental health issue and subsequently be admitted to hospital than their white British counterparts. BME groups are more likely than white British counterparts to have a poorer treatment outcome from a period of inpatient care and are more likely to disengage from mainstream health services, leading to social exclusion and a decline in their mental health. In the UK patients from BME groups are also more likely to be detained under a section of the *Mental Health Act 1983* (Singh *et al.* 2007).

The reasons for these observed differences may be manifold, but poverty and racism are thought to be key factors. Crucially, though, it is argued that contemporary health services (including mental health services) do not understand or cater for non-white British communities and fail to meet the cultural needs of other populations.

Implications for practice

It could be argued that many mental health problems go unreported/untreated in minority ethnic populations. It is important to recognise that some minority groups understand mental health and British mental health services differently. For example, a Rastafarian person may smoke cannabis as part of their cultural and spiritual identity; similarly a Somalian person may chew khat as part of their social custom. However, the types of mental health issues are likely to be the same, with people experiencing:

- anxiety and depression;
- psychosis and schizophrenia;

- substance misuse;
- bipolar disorder;
- personality disorder.

The role of the mental health nurse

The role of mental health nurse when working with culturally and ethnically diverse people and communities includes:

- challenging stigma and racism;
- seeking to understand cultural differences;
- offering supportive counselling;
- encouraging links with social and ethnic groups;
- offering medication as prescribed;
- offering interpreters and advocates when possible.

Homelessness

Background

Homelessness is an extreme form of social exclusion and attracts significant health issues. There is an increasing body of evidence of a significantly higher rate of mental health issues amongst the homeless adult population than the population with homes and shelter (QNI 2012).

Reports suggest that the incidence of psychosis and substance misuse is considerably higher amongst the homeless population, and yet the homeless are amongst the least able members of society to access health care (Melvin 2004). Many homeless individuals, rough sleepers and those living in hostels and insecure accommodation are either not registered with a general practitioner (GP), or find it difficult to do so. Access to secondary care services is therefore even more difficult for people experiencing serious mental illness because a referral from a GP is often required. Homeless people therefore utilise accident and emergency services, which is inappropriate and costly.

Implications for practice

Reports suggest that homeless adults experience twice the rate of neurotic disorder (anxiety and depression) than the general population. Other mental health conditions experienced by homeless adults are listed below:

- substance misuse;
- schizophrenia and psychosis;
- bipolar disorder;
- self-harm;
- personality disorder.

Social isolation and stigma can pose significant barriers to interventions from mental health professionals. Previous poor experience from mental health services may also make homeless people reluctant to engage. Liaison and collaboration with dedicated homeless workers is key to engagement; as is registration with a general practitioner.

The role of the mental health nurse
The role of the mental health nurse when working with people who are homeless includes:

- working with dedicated worker who work with homeless populations;
- encouraging concordance with prescribed medication;
- discouraging alcohol/substance misuse;
- encouraging sleep hygiene;
- offering cognitive behavioural therapy to assist with anxiety;
- encouraging healthy eating and regular exercise;
- signposting the homeless adult to social groups and encourage positive relationships;
- assisting with housing, where possible;
- engaging with a community mental health worker, as required.

Older adults

Background
A decline in mental health is not a symptom of aging. Indeed, many older adults live full, active and mentally well lives. That said, the older adult is as likely as a younger adult to experience a mental health issue (Parker 2012). The incidence of depression, however, is higher amongst older people, with factors such as retirement, bereavement, physical disability and loneliness contributing to the condition (Parker 2012). Mental ill health amongst older people is often further compounded by physical co-morbidity; conditions such as heart disease, respiratory disease, reduced mobility and other chronic conditions inevitably impact upon mental health. In addition to depression, common mental health conditions amongst older adults include:

- dementia;
- delirium;
- alcohol abuse.

Implications for practice
Dementia is a condition that affects predominantly older people, and advancing age is a risk factor for development of the disease. Dementia is a progressive, degenerative disease, characterised by a decline in cognitive function resulting in changes to a person's memory, thinking,

orientation and personality. The National Dementia Strategy (DoH 2009) fosters a philosophy of living well with dementia, however, the needs of a person living with dementia will inevitably change as the condition progresses. Furthermore, a high proportion of those living with dementia will experience depression, which, for some, may be undiagnosed.

Delirium is a common condition amongst older people and results in a rapid decline in cognitive function coupled with confusion. It can be caused by infection, medication, poor nutrition, constipation, alcohol consumption and dehydration. It is an urgent medical condition, but the symptoms are easily reversible, usually requiring the underlying cause to be addressed, and sometimes this is as simple as a course of antibiotics.

Alcohol use amongst older adults is not uncommon and can be a serious health risk, not only because abrupt cessation can induce delirium but also because the older adult is more sensitive to the effects of alcohol. Excessive alcohol consumption can lead to falls and accidents, and a decline in mental health, causing conditions such as depression and anxiety.

The role of the mental health nurse

The role of mental health nurse when working with older adults includes:

- ensuring that depression is diagnosed and treated;
- offering psychological interventions and therapies;
- supporting medication adherence;
- signposting to appropriate financial and welfare services;
- ensuring physiological well-being and pain are managed;
- encouraging physical activity and a good diet;
- encouraging contact with social groups or condition-specific groups;
- working collaboratively with carers;
- preserving dignity and respect;
- collaborating with alcohol services and offering psychoeducation.

Safeguarding vulnerable adults

Background

A vulnerable adult is defined as being 'aged 18 years or over…who is or may be in need of community care services by reason of mental or other disability, age or illness; and who is or may be unable to take care of him or herself, or unable to protect him or herself from significant harm or exploitation' (DoH 2000). A vulnerable adult is not restricted to any specific gender, diagnosis or strata of society but may include:

- an older person;
- a person with a learning disability;
- a person with dementia;

- a person with a mental health issue;
- a person with a long-term health condition;
- person who abuses substances.

Abuse is about the misuse of power and is based on the principle of whether harm was *caused* rather than whether harm was *intended*. Simply failing to act to prevent harm can, by definition, be classed as abuse. Abuse can take many forms and can take place in many settings, including care homes, residential homes, hospitals, clinics and educational establishments. Typically, abuse is classed as:

- physical abuse;
- emotional abuse;
- sexual abuse;
- neglect and acts of omission;
- financial abuse;
- discriminatory abuse;
- institutional abuse.

Note that there is likely to be some overlap; for example, if a person is being sexually abused they may well be physically and emotionally abused at the same time.

Implications for practice

Safeguarding is everyone's business, although responsibilities for it will vary depending on role and responsibilities. According the Social Care Institute for Excellence (SCIE 2014), the key principles of adult protection are:

- empowerment — presumption of person-led decisions and informed consent;
- protection — support and representation for those in greatest need;
- prevention — it is better to take action before harm occurs;
- proportionality — use the most proportionate and least intrusive response appropriate to the risk presented;
- partnership — seek local solutions by working with communities (communities have a part to play in preventing, detecting and reporting neglect and abuse);
- accountability — ensure accountability and transparency in delivering safeguarding.

Further to this, the *Care Act 2014* outlines a clear legal framework for how local authorities and agencies in the UK should protect adults at risk of abuse of neglect. Under this act, local authorities have specific safeguarding duties, including promoting multi-agency working, establishing local adult safeguarding boards, carrying out safeguarding reviews and arranging for advocacy when appropriate.

The role of the mental health nurse

All mental health nurses are duty-bound to safeguard the people in their care and follow the appropriate policies and legal frameworks that assist the safeguarding of vulnerable adults. It is vital that local policies and procedures are followed, and when there are concerns about risk and safety the alarm is raised, concerns are expressed, escalated and recorded, and appropriate action is taken. When a person discloses abuse it is important to:

- stay calm;
- tell the person that you will have to share the information (under a confidentiality statement);
- listen carefully;
- not ask direct or leading questions;
- encourage but don't pressurise;
- make detailed notes;
- do not contact the suspected abuser or commence covert surveillance;
- keep the details confidential, according to organisational policy.

As mental health nurses it is imperative to maintain confidentiality while at the same time sharing appropriate information with the appropriate agencies. It goes without saying that disclosures should be handled sensitively, respectfully and supportively in a non-judgmental way.

Sexual abuse

Background

Child sexual abuse involves forcing or enticing a child to take part in sexual activities whether or not the child is aware of what's happening (HMG 2015). There are two types of child sex abuse: contact abuse and non-contact abuse. Contact abuse is when an abuser makes physical contact with the child and non-contact abuse is when the abuser does not touch the child, but persuades the child to perform sexual acts. According to the National Society for the Prevention of Cruelty to Children (NSPCC 2015) child sex abuse involves:

- sexual touching (with or without clothes on) including kissing, rubbing, masturbating or using an object;
- sexual penetration, including rape or penetration of the mouth, with a part of the body or an object;
- encouraging a child to take part in sexual activity, such as having sex or masturbating;
- not taking the correct measures to protect a child from sexual exploitation;
- meeting a child following sexual grooming;

- taking, making, showing or distributing indecent images of children;
- paying for the sexual services of a child;
- encouraging a child to engage in prostitution or pornography;
- showing a child images of sexual activity, including photos, videos or via a webcam.

Note that sexual abuse is not the sole proclivity of men; woman can abuse children as can other children.

Implications for practice

It is not clear why people sexually abuse children, but the relationship between child sex abuse and the development of mental health issues in childhood and adult life is well accepted in the literature (Mullen *et al.* 1993). Studies have shown that victims of sexual abuse are four times more likely to have increased contact with mental health services than the general population (Spataro *et al.* 2004). Conditions across the whole mental health spectrum are reported, but the conditions listed below are thought to be more prevalent:

- post-traumatic stress disorder;
- depression;
- suicide;
- substance abuse.

Some studies suggest that there is a link between child sexual abuse and the development of schizophrenia and personality disorder (Spataro *et al.*2004). However, these studies are limited and most studies are confined to female populations.

The role of the mental health nurse

The mental health needs of those who have been sexually abused require a sensitive, empathic and non-judgmental therapeutic approach. If a service user discloses sexual abuse, it is important that the mental health nurse can then manage that disclosure. Depending on their specific expertise and role, a mental health nurse may offer the following:

- antidepressant medication;
- talking therapies (counselling);
- cognitive behavioural therapy;
- psychodynamic therapy;
- group therapy and self-help.

Sexuality and gender

Background

Being lesbian, gay, bisexual or transgender (LGBT) is not a mental illness in itself, despite having previously been labelled as such. However, it is likely that many LGBT people will experience more mental health issues compared to their heterosexual counterparts (King *et al.* 2008); in fact, depression and anxiety are common conditions amongst this group. Higher incidences of depression and anxiety may have resulted from the experience of being LGBT in a largely heterosexist and transphobic society. It is likely that individuals may have experienced rejection, stigma, prejudice and social exclusion from society, family members and health professionals, which may damage their self-esteem and further compound their mental ill health.

Implications for practice

It not uncommon for a LGBT person to struggle with their sexuality and to hide it from their family, friends, mental health professionals and colleagues, and in some cases lead a double life. Furthermore, the LGBT person may well have experienced discrimination and prejudice from health providers when attempting to access support and services. Studies suggest that this prejudice can take the form of homophobic comments from health professionals and escalating to health professionals making links between the service user's sexuality and their mental health condition (DoH 2007a). This can cause unnecessary mental anguish, leading to:

- depression;
- anxiety;
- deliberate self-harm and suicide attempts;
- drug and alcohol misuse;
- post-traumatic stress disorder.

Factors such as age, religion and ethnicity can further complicate mental distress.

The role of the mental health nurse

The health needs of the LGBT population can be quite specific and so it is vital that providers of care are able to sensitively discuss issues around sex and sexuality in an empathic, person-centred way that is non-judgmental and anti-discriminatory. Note that it is illegal under the *Equality Act 2010* to discriminate against someone on the grounds of their sexual orientation. Depending on their expertise and experience, mental health nurses may offer or deliver:

- psychotherapy;
- counselling;
- talking therapies;
- cognitive behavioural therapy;
- pink therapy and LGBT-specific psychotherapy;
- antidepressant medication;
- anxiolytic medication.

Spirituality and religion

Background

Spirituality means different things to different people. Although it is traditionally expressed through various forms of art, nature and built environments, more modern approaches to spirituality have become varied and accepted (MHF 2007). Common themes that describe spirituality include:

- a search for hope or harmony;
- a belief in a higher being or beings;
- a level of transcendence, or the sense that there is more to life than the material or practical;

Although spirituality differs from conventional religious traditions, many religions have their own distinct community-based worship, beliefs, sacred texts and traditions in which spirituality is incorporated. Spirituality and religion may of course be related, but not necessarily synonymous. Spirituality can add meaning to the practice of religion, for instance, and the practice of religion can deepen spirituality (Adams et al. 2000). Every person can have their own unique experience of spirituality, with or without a traditional religious belief (RCP 2014).

Implications for practice

Religion may, for some, provide answers to fundamental life questions. It may also help young people to form their personal identity (Schwartz et al. 2013). Studies on Islam and mental health using Muslim participants have reached the conclusions that there is a positive relationship between religiosity and both mental health and subjective well-being, and a negative association between religiosity and psychopathology (Abdel-Khalek, 2011). Satori (2010) suggests that due to a lack of practical guidance nurses are often unsure on how to meet a patient's spiritual needs.

The role of the mental health nurse

Baker and Cruickshank (2009) suggest that there is great value to combining religious activities in treatment and recovery for patients who are Muslim, with patients feeling this is as effective as any medication. Within Western clinical settings, professionals perhaps underestimate the importance of a patient's spirituality and how a person's religious practice affects care and personal engagement (Phelps et al. 2012). The Nursing and Midwifery Council developed a strategy (NMC 2015) that encompasses race, religion, culture and ethnicity. The strategy uses the Equality Act 2010 as a guide to how nurses should conduct themselves when treating patients who belong to different religious and cultural backgrounds. The NMC aims to develop nurses' understanding of different ethnic backgrounds through education and training and put an emphasis on professionals valuing the importance of diversity (NMC 2015).

LIBRARY, UNIVERSITY OF CHESTER

Appendices

Anatomy and physiology

Background

The human body is a complex structure that consists of different systems that constantly interact with each other. We will describe each system separately; however, it has to be acknowledged that when all these systems work effectively together the body maintains a healthy state. In keeping with a *Rapid* book this section provides an overview of each system, highlighting the main features, rather than providing the detail you would expect to find in a dedicated anatomy and physiology text. In this section, the systems of the body are ordered to start with the outer-facing part of the body, the skin, followed by the structural framework of the body, the bones and muscles, and concluding with the body's internal systems. Building on an overview of the human body, this section will then highlight the clinical procedures that mental health nurses need to be proficient in. These procedures as whole assist the nurse in the process of monitoring a service user's vital signs.

Skin

Although skin is not usually described as a body system it is worth mentioning here as it is the largest organ of the body. Skin has three main parts: the epidermis, the thin outer layer of the skin; the dermis, the middle layer of the skin that includes hair follicles, sweat glands, nerve fibres, and lymphatic and blood vessels; and the hypodermis, where fat is stored.

Functions of the skin:

- to protect the body against harmful microorganisms and foreign material;
- to prevent excessive fluid loss from the body;
- to help regulate the temperature of the body;
- to synthesise vitamin D;
- to assist the process of excretion;
- to help the body to perceive heat, cold, touch, pressure and pain (sensory reception).

The skeletal system

The skeletal system is composed of bones, cartilages and ligaments. Structurally, the skeletal system provides attachment points for the body's muscles; it also provides movement through a series of joints.

Rapid Mental Health Nursing, First Edition. Grahame Smith and Rebecca Rylance.
© 2016 John Wiley & Sons, Ltd. Published 2016 by John Wiley & Sons, Ltd.

Functions of the skeletal system:

- to provide an internal and stable framework upon which the rest of body grows;
- to support, protect and anchor the body's organs;
- to store essential minerals, such as calcium, phosphorus and iron;
- to assist with the production of new blood cells via the bone marrow.

The muscular system

Muscles can be skeletal, cardiac or smooth. Skeletal muscles are part of the musculoskeletal system, for example the triceps muscle in the arm, and can be moved by conscious thought (voluntary). Cardiac muscles can be moved by conscious thought, albeit in a limited way (involuntary). Smooth muscles, for example the tissue within the bladder tissue of the intestines, are completely involuntary and cannot be moved by conscious thought.

Functions of the muscular system:

- to work with the skeletal system to provide strength, stability and posture;
- to enable a full range of movement, both external and internal movement;
- to generate heat to keep the body warm.

The nervous system

The nervous system is one of the body's communication and control systems (the other is the endocrine system). It is comprised of two main parts: the central nervous system, which includes the brain and the spinal cord; and the peripheral nervous system, which includes the nerve fibres that branch out from the central nervous system to all parts of the body. The peripheral nervous system can be divided into three parts: the autonomic, which controls involuntary actions; the sensory, which provides sensory information to the central nervous system; and motor, which transmits signals from the brain to the skeletal muscles.

Functions of the nervous system:

- to help coordinate the body's voluntary and involuntary movements;
- to transmit electrical and chemical signals to and from different parts of the body.

The endocrine system

The endocrine system is the second of the body's communication and control systems. It is important to note that both the nervous and endocrine systems work together to enable all the other body systems to work in unison. The endocrine system consists of hormone-producing glands, which secrete hormones into the bloodstream to enable the body to transmit information to various parts of the body. The hormone-producing glands include the pineal, pituitary, thyroid, parathyroid and adrenal glands. The pancreas, ovaries, testes hypothalamus and the gastrointestinal tract also play a central part in this system.

Functions of the endocrine system:

- to enable the body to control and regulate body functions including growth, metabolism and sexual reproduction;
- to control the body's slow processes, such as cell development.

The cardiovascular system

The cardiovascular system carries blood around the body and consists of the heart and a network of blood vessels, such as arteries, veins and capillaries. The heart drives or pumps blood around the body and the blood vessels provide a means by which blood can travel to and from the heart. Blood is composed of cells and plasma (fluid). Three main types of blood cells are: white blood cells, which help to fight infection; red blood cells, which can carry oxygen; and platelets, which are part of the body's clotting mechanism and aim to prevent blood loss.

Functions of the cardiovascular system:

- to transport oxygen and nutrients to all parts of body;
- to remove waste material from body tissues;
- to help the body fight infection.

The respiratory system

The respiratory system provides oxygen, which is needed to convert food into energy, to the body. Air consists primarily of oxygen, nitrogen and carbon dioxide and is inhaled through the nasal passages and into the lungs. Oxygen is then exchanged with carbon dioxide, which then leaves the blood to be exhaled into the outside air, and the oxygen is then transported to the body's cells. The respiratory system is composed of the nasal cavities, pharynx, larynx, trachea and the lungs.

Functions of the respiratory system:

- to supply oxygen to the body;
- to remove carbon dioxide from the body.

The digestive system

The digestive system breaks down food (digestion) into components small enough to be used by the body's cells (absorption). These processes enable the body to extract essential nutrients from food; any food that is not used is then eliminated from the body. As food is being broken down it is moved through the digestive system through a process of peristalsis (muscular contractions). Digestive organs include the mouth, pharynx, oesophagus, stomach, intestines, rectum and the anus.

Functions of the digestive system:

- to break down food into essential nutrients that are easy to absorb;
- to eliminate food waste from the body.

The urinary system

The urinary system works as a filtering system, removing waste products from blood and then excreting residual waste products from the body (as urine). The urinary system consists of the kidneys, ureters, bladder and the urethra. Urine is stored in the bladder and is then expelled from the body through the urethra.

Functions of the urinary system:

- to filter waste products from the blood;
- to excrete urine;
- to regulate the volume and pressure of blood within the body;
- to control the levels of electrolytes (salts and minerals) and other substances within the body;
- to regulate blood pH to ensure it is not too acidic or alkaline.

Clinical procedures

Blood glucose

The purpose of this procedure is to measure the amount of glucose in the blood, which is expressed as millimoles per litre (mmol/L); the normal range is between 4–8 mmol/L.

Equipment required
- a calibrated blood glucose meter/monitor;
- blood glucose test strips that are in date and have not been contaminated;
- single-use lancets and lancet device;
- gloves;
- cotton wool or gauze;
- sharps box.

Procedure
First of all the nurse will explain the procedure to the service user and obtain their consent. Then the nurse will:

- ask the service user to ether sit or lie down;
- wash hands and put on gloves;
- insert a clean lancet into the lancet device;
- take a blood sample from the side of the finger, using an appropriate lancet depth and remembering to rotate the piercing site;
- apply a drop of blood to the correct part of the testing strip;
- place the strip in the meter/monitor if this is not required before taking a sample of blood;

- dispose of the lancet in the sharps box;
- place the cotton wool or gauze over the puncture site and apply gentle pressure if required; monitor for excessive bleeding;
- follow the directions on the meter/monitor to obtain a reading;
- wash hands;
- document the results and report any unexpected readings, errors or excessive bleeding.

Blood pressure

The purpose of this procedure is to measure the pressure of blood against the vessel walls. The usual site for measuring blood pressure is the brachial artery in the upper arm. Blood pressure can be measured manually or automatically, using a machine. Normal blood pressure is measured in millimetres of mercury (mmHg) and can range from 110–140 mmHg for systolic pressure and from 70–80 mmHg for diastolic pressure.

Equipment required
- an appropriately sized cuff;
- a calibrated sphygmomanometer;
- a stethoscope;
- a chair with an arm rest or equivalent;
- detergent hand wipes.

Procedure
First of all the nurse will explain the procedure to the service user and obtain their consent. Then the nurse will:

- wash hands;
- check if the service user has a preference for using a particular arm;
- ensure the service user is seated and rests for three to five minutes before having their blood pressure measured. The service user should not be eating, drinking or talking when their blood pressure measurement is taken;
- ensure that the upper arm is supported and positioned at heart level, and is free from clothing. The sphygmomanometer should be no more than a meter away from the nurse and it should be at eye level;
- wrap the cuff around the arm, ensuring that the centre of the bladder covers the brachial artery;
- inflate the cuff while palpating the brachial artery; when the pulse can no longer be felt the nurse will inflate the cuff rapidly for a further 20–30 mmHg;
- deflate the cuff until the pulse reappears, note the reading and then deflate the cuff;

- after 15–20 seconds place the diaphragm of the stethoscope over the brachial artery; note that the diaphragm of the stethoscope should not be tucked under the edge of the cuff.

Peak flow rate

The purpose of this procedure is to measure the 'maximum flow of air which can be achieved when air is expired with maximum force following maximum inspiration' (Dougherty and Lister 2011: 745). Peak flow is measured by comparing the volume of air a person breathes out (litres per minute, L/min) against what would be expected for a person of that age. The normal limit for men is up to 100 L/min lower than predicted for age and he normal limit for women is 85 L/min lower than predicted for age.

Equipment required

- a calibrated peak flow meter;
- a disposable mouthpiece.

Procedure

First of all the nurse will explain the procedure to the service user and obtain their consent. Then the nurse will:

- wash hands;
- assemble the peak flow meter with a clean mouthpiece;
- ask the service user to adopt a comfortable position, either sitting or standing. The same position should be used for all future readings;
- set the pointer on the scale to zero;
- ask the service user to hold the peak flow meter horizontally;
- ask the service user to take a deep breath (full inspiration) through their mouth;
- ask the service user to place their lips tightly around the mouthpiece, ensuring a good seal. The inspiration should not be held for longer than two seconds;
- ask the service user to breathe out as hard and as fast as possible;
- note the reading, and then ask the service user to repeat the procedure twice;
- document the results and report any unexpected or abnormal readings;
- dispose the mouthpiece and clean the meter;
- wash hands.

Pulse

The purpose of this procedure is to count the pulse, which is equivalent to measuring heart rate. A normal pulse rate for a healthy adult is between 60 and 100 beats per minute. The pulse can be felt in any place that enables an artery to be compressed against a bone, such as the neck, wrist, knee, inside of the elbow and near the ankle joint. The pulse is usually taken at the wrist — the radial site, and not only is the rate noted but also the rhythm and amplitude (pulse strength). The nurse measures the pulse by 'lightly compressing the artery against firm tissue and by counting the number of beats per minute' (Dougherty and Lister, 2011: 708).

Equipment required
- a watch with a second hand;
- alcohol hand rub.

Procedure
First of all the nurse will explain the procedure to the service user and obtain their consent. Then the nurse will:

- wash hands;
- ensure the service user is comfortable and has refrained from physical activity for 20 minutes prior to their pulse being taken;
- place the first and second finger along the artery and apply light pressure until the pulse is felt;
- count the pulse (the number of beats) for 60 seconds;
- wash hands;
- document the results and report any unexpected readings.

Respiratory rate
The purpose of this procedure is to assess the:

- airway — checking for obstructions;
- breathing — rate, rhythm and depth;
- skin colour — looking for cyanosis (a blue tone to the skin);
- use of accessory muscles — looking for breathing through flared nostrils or pursed lips;
- general condition — level of consciousness.

Equipment required
- a watch with a second hand.

Procedure
First of all the nurse will explain the procedure to the service user and obtain their consent. Then the nurse will:

- ensure the service user is comfortable;
- monitor and record the service user's respirations immediately after taking the pulse to avoid the service user altering their breathing;

- observe the rise (inspiration) and fall (expiration) of the chest for one breath;
- count the service user's respirations for 60 seconds;
- note the pattern of breathing and the depth of the service user's breath;
- document the results and report any unexpected readings.

Temperature

The purpose of this procedure is to measure a service user's temperature. Normal temperature is in the range 36.0–37.2°C. Temperature can be measured at a number of sites; however the development of new technology means that it is now more common to measure temperature via the tympanic membrane (ear canal).

Equipment required

- tympanic membrane thermometer;
- disposable probe covers;
- alcohol hand rub.

Procedure

First of all the nurse will explain the procedure to the service user and obtain their consent. Then the nurse will:

- wash hands;
- ensure good access to the service user's ear and document which ear is being used to ensure consistency of results;
- apply the disposable cover to the probe;
- place the probe gently into the ear;
- measure the temperature and record the reading;
- dispose of the probe cover;
- wash hands;
- document the results and report any unexpected readings.

Urinalysis

The purpose of this procedure is to analyse the composition of a service user's urine by using a dipstick test. A strip coated with chemicals is dipped into urine and the results are compared to the manufacturer's guidelines on the bottle or container.

Equipment required

- gloves;
- apron;
- urine dipsticks that are in date and have not been contaminated;
- urine specimen bottle;

Procedure

First of all the nurse will explain the procedure to the service user and obtain their consent. Then the nurse will:

- wash hands and put on gloves and apron;
- collect a clean and fresh specimen of urine;
- remove the dipstick and immediately replace the cap on the container;
- immerse the dipstick into urine and wait for the appropriate length of time (following manufacturer's instructions);
- run the edge of the strip against the rim of the specimen bottle to remove any excess urine;
- hold the dipstick at a slight angle, preventing pad-to-pad contamination;
- after waiting the required length of time (following manufacturer's instructions) compare the strip against the reference guide on the dipstick container;
- dispose of urine and dipstick;
- remove gloves and apron;
- wash hands;
- document the results and report any abnormal readings.

Revision questions

Each question has one correct answer.

Essential skills and knowledge

1. Which of the following accurately describes the assessment and care-delivery process?
   a) Assessment, care delivery, care planning and goal setting, and evaluation
   b) Assessment, care planning and goal setting, care delivery, and evaluation
   c) Assessment, care planning and goal setting, evaluation and care delivery
   d) Assessment, care delivery, evaluation, and care planning and goal setting

2. Which of the following is a mental-health-specific nursing model?
   a) King's open systems model
   b) Neuman's systems model
   c) Orem's self-care model
   d) Peplau's interpersonal relations model
   e) Roy's adaptation model

3. Which of the following influences the decision-making process?
   a) Identifying the issue
   b) Analysing the evidence
   c) Asking "What are you trying to achieve?"
   d) Critiquing different forms of evidence
   e) Delivering the chosen intervention

4. Which of the following is not a clinical observation?
   a) Peak flow rate
   b) Pulse
   c) Respiration
   d) Intramuscular injection
   e) Temperature
   f) Blood pressure

Rapid Mental Health Nursing, First Edition. Grahame Smith and Rebecca Rylance.
© 2016 John Wiley & Sons, Ltd. Published 2016 by John Wiley & Sons, Ltd.

5. Which risk-assessment approach uses evidence-based research to influence the types of risk information collected?
   a) Unstructured risk assessment
   b) Actuarial risk assessent
   c) Clinical risk assessment
   d) Structured risk assessment

6. Which of the following is not one of the 6C's?
   a) Care
   b) Courage
   c) Consideration
   d) Competence
   e) Communication

7. Classifying mental illnesses aims to provide a framework that improves:
   a) The diagnostic process, communication and treatment outcomes
   b) Assessment, treatment and control
   c) The diagnostic process, treatment and risk management
   d) Risk management, control and treatment

8. When reflecting on their record-keeping what should a mental health nurse consider?
   a) Have you documented everything that happened during the shift?
   b) Does your entry provide accurate evidence of the standard of care delivered?
   c) Is your opinion included?
   d) Does your entry provide accurate evidence of the care delivered?

9. When a person is considered to be at risk of developing a psychosis they should be offered:
   a) Mindfulness work and systemic family therapy
   b) Individual cognitive behavioural therapy with or without family intervention or other interventions in accordance with agreed clinical guidelines
   c) Antipsychotic medication and family interventions
   d) Individual behavioural therapy, family therapy and antipsychotic medication

10. Electroconvulsive therapy is not contraindicated in:
   a) Raised intracranial pressure
   b) Cardiovascular disease
   c) Dementias
   d) Epilepsy
   e) Depression

11. Which of the following describes overflow incontinence?
    a) A leakage of urine that usually happens during physical activity
    b) An uncontrollable urge to pass urine and at times an individual may find it difficult to make it to the toilet in time
    c) An individual uncontrollably passes small amounts of urine during the day and night
    d) A complete leakage of urine without the individual having a feeling of needing to go to the toilet or having control

12. Which of the following is not a consistent infection-control practice:
    a) Receiving training on the standard principles of effective infection control and prevention
    b) Adhering to local and national reporting procedures for infections
    c) Managing and monitoring the prevention and control of infection using a robust risk-assessment process
    d) Providing a comfortable and secure care environment
    e) Providing user-friendly and accurate information on infections and infection control

13. Which theory or model of leadership focuses on enhancing the performance of individuals?
    a) Traits-based
    b) Behavioural
    c) Situational-contingency
    d) Transformational

14. The two Prep standards are:
    a) Preceptor and continuing professional development standards
    b) Practice and continuing professional development standards
    c) Practice and lifelong learning standards
    d) Continuing professional development and expert practice standards

15. Which of the following is not a factor behind incidents of violence and aggression that occur in inpatient mental health settings?
    a) The service user being highly impulsive
    b) Poor staff attitudes and behaviours — especially poor communication skills
    c) Accessible staff
    d) Locked wards
    e) Lack of privacy for service users

16. Which of the following is not a common management function?
    a) Managing performance
    b) Delegation

c) Agreeing lunch breaks
d) Managing change
e) Decision-making

17. When managing risk the mental health nurse should consider which of the following?
a) Control all risks
b) Report incidents only when they arise
c) Recognise only self-harm and harm to other
d) Be aware of the potential risks of the care they deliver
e) Manage risk as an independent part of practice

18. Which of the following is an anti-dementia medication?
a) Donepezil
b) Chlorpromazine
c) Risperidone
d) Quetiapine
e) Haloperidol

19. In relation to the management of medication a mental health nurse is professionally required to:
a) Ensure that managing medicines is built on safe and effective practice which is underpinned by a commitment to work in partnership
b) Administer medicines in keeping with an inpatient setting's internal practices
c) Keep and maintain records that are in accordance with their own standards
d) Ensure that their medicine management practice adheres only to local policy guidelines

20. Which civil section of the *Mental Health Act 1983 (amended 2007)* has a duration of 28 days?
a) Section 3
b) Section 35
c) Section 2
d) Section 5.2

21. When assessing nutritional intake which of the following information should you collect?
a) Height only
b) Waist-to-hip ratio
c) Physical appearance only
d) Dietary intake over the last six hours
e) Eating difficulties only

22. What is a common approach that mental health nurses will use to organise care within community mental health settings?
    a) Service-user allocation
    b) Task approach
    c) Team nursing approach
    d) Case management approach
    e) Primary nursing approach

23. A physical health assessment for individuals with mental health needs should include:
    a) Physical health information, a physical examination and baseline investigations
    b) Physical health information, a physical examination and blood tests
    c) A physical examination and investigations, including include blood tests
    d) Medical history, a neurological examination and blood tests

24. Which of following are the two distinct parts of a psychiatric examination?
    a) The psychiatric history and mental state examination
    b) The mental state examination including formulation
    c) The psychiatric history and mental state examination including formulation
    d) The psychiatric history and formulation

25. In terms of psychological interventions mental health nurses are professionally required to:
    a) Focus on controlling risky individuals
    b) Prevent social isolation and promote social functioning
    c) Focus on early warning signs and the self-monitoring of symptoms
    d) Be person centred and committed to building therapeutic relationships that are enabling and partnership focused
    e) Be trained as cognitive behavioural therapists

26. Eye movement desensitisation and reprocessing is a treatment used in which mental health condition?
    a) Depression
    b) Psychosis
    c) Post-traumatic stress disorder
    d) Obsessive compulsive disorder
    e) Eating disorders

27. Which recovery model has three key components or domains?
    a) Tidal model
    b) Collaborative recovery model
    c) Strengths model
    d) Well-being and recovery action plan approach

28. Reflection on action is:
    a) Identifying and describing an experience
    b) Examining the experience in depth
    c) Reflecting after an experience and then taking action to improve practice
    d) Reflecting during the experience so that previous learning is used to improve practice

29. Generally, which form of research focuses on measuring and cause and effect?
    a) Qualitative
    b) Phenomenology
    c) Quantitative
    d) Ethnography
    e) Interviews

30. Deliberate self-harm is:
    a) Trying to kill oneself and not succeeding; it may or may not be intentional, it may be a suicidal gesture, a cry for help or an act of revenge
    b) Intentionally injuring oneself; there may or may not be suicidal intent
    c) Intentionally killing oneself
    d) Intentionally trying to kill oneself and not succeeding

31. Which of the following is an essential element of the therapeutic relationship?
    a) Being focused
    b) Having all the answers
    c) Being empathetic
    d) Being persuasive
    e) Being unemotional

32. When delegating what do you have to consider?
    a) Who is accountable and responsible?
    b) Does the person do as they are told?
    c) Can they do the task quickly?
    d) Would it be less hassle if you completed the task instead?

33. Which following ethical theory is primarily concerned with outcomes?
    a) Deontology
    b) Consequentialism
    c) Virtues-based ethics
    d) Principlism

Conditions

1. If a person is diagnosed with delirium and they are quiet and withdrawn the type of delirium could be:
   a) Hyperactive delirium
   b) Hypoactive delirium
   c) Dementia
   d) Mixed delirium

2. Hazardous drinking is when:
   a) Men consume 10–30 units and women 15–35 units weekly
   b) Men consume 22–50 units and women 5–20 units weekly
   c) Men consume over 50 units and women over 35 units weekly
   d) Men consume 22–50 units and women 15–35 units weekly
   e) Men consume over 50 units and women 15–35 units weekly

3. Generalised anxiety disorder is:
   a) Recurrent and severe panic attacks that occur unpredictably
   b) A generalised and persistent anxiety lasting at least longer than three weeks
   c) Fear which can become panic of specific situations, places, objects, animals, heights and closed or open spaces
   d) Recurrent obsessional thoughts or compulsive acts with a frequency greater than one hour per day and with duration of at least two weeks

4. Rapid cycling is a type of which condition?
   a) Schizophrenia
   b) Depression
   c) Delirium
   d) Bipolar affective disorder

5. Overdosing on what is the most common known method of self-harm in adolescents?
   a) Paracetamol
   b) Aspirin
   c) Methadone
   d) Antidepressants

6. Which syndrome is categorised by multiple cognitive impairments including memory, orientation, language, comprehension, and reasoning?
   a) Bipolar affective disorder
   b) Schizophrenia
   c) Dementia
   d) Delirium

7. Which condition are the symptoms of low mood, loss of interest and low energy primarily associated with?
   a) Personality disorder
   b) Schizophrenia
   c) Depression
   d) Anxiety
   e) Substance misuse

8. In cases of extreme fear of childbirth it is essential to do what?
   a) Deliver low-intensity psychological interventions only
   b) Deliver psychological interventions and involve the wider perinatal team
   c) Deliver high-intensity psychological interventions only
   d) Deliver psychological interventions and administer medication

9. Illicit drugs can generally be divided into which of the following categories?
   a) Opiates, stimulants, hallucinogens and cannabis
   b) Opiates, stimulants and hallucinogens
   c) Stimulants, hallucinogens and cannabis
   d) Opiates, stimulants, hallucinogens, cannabis and alcohol

10. Exercise and nutritional education are psychological interventions in which condition?
    a) Depression
    b) Personality disorder
    c) Eating disorders
    d) Delirium
    e) Bipolar affective disorder

11. Older adults are less likely to report
    a) Aggression
    b) Low mood or suicidal thoughts
    c) Irritability
    d) Financial difficulties

12. The prevalence of individuals with a learning disability in the general population in the UK is approximately:
    a) 5%
    b) 3%
    c) 10%
    d) 1.5%

13. Neuropsychiatry divides mental disorders attributable to diseases of the nervous system into how many types?
    a) Four
    b) Five
    c) Two
    d) Three

14. Which condition is categorised by clusters and types?
    a) Schizophrenia
    b) Obsessive compulsive disorder
    c) Personality disorder
    d) Mild cognitive impairment

15. The term schizophrenia means:
    a) Split mind
    b) Split personality
    c) Disordered mind
    d) Unreal mind

16. Sexual disorder is?
    a) Abnormal sexual functioning
    b) The impairment of normal sexual functioning
    c) Low sex drive
    d) High sex drive

17. Persistent sleep disorders can often lead to:
    a) Dementia
    b) Personality disorders
    c) Anxiety and depression
    d) Obsessive compulsive disorder

18. Reactive attachment disorder is:
    a) A child withdraws emotionally from social contact due to abuse,
       neglect etc.
    b) A stressor, such as distress at work and/or home, leads to anxiety
       and/or depression longer than you expect for most people
    c) A child becomes unreserved in their interactions with
       unfamiliar adults due to abuse, neglect etc.
    d) A fearful response to threatening and/or catastrophic event

19. Unresolved grief is where grief is:
    a) Less than 6 months after the death of a close other, delayed in
       onset and more intense than you would normally expect to see
    b) Prolonged beyond 6 months after the death of a close other,
       delayed in onset and more intense than you would normally
       expect to see
    c) Prolonged beyond 6 months after the death of a close other,
       sudden onset and more intense than you would normally
       expect to see
    d) Prolonged beyond 6 months after the death of a close other,
       delayed in onset and less intense than you would normally
       expect to see

Specific issues

1. When a refugee has had their claim for protection approved by the government this is known as:
   a) Asylum
   b) Leave to remain
   c) Nationalisation
   d) Citizenship

2. Generally speaking, black people and minority ethnic groups are more likely to be:
   a) Diagnosed with a mental health issue and subsequently be admitted to hospital than their white British counterparts
   b) Diagnosed with a mental health issue and subsequently treated in the community than their white British counterparts
   c) Diagnosed with a mental health issue and subsequently be admitted to hospital at the same rate as their white British counterparts
   d) Not diagnosed with a mental health issue and not access mental health services

3. Homelessness is:
   a) A form of social exclusion; however, it attracts no significant health issues
   b) Not a form of social exclusion; however, it attracts significant health issues
   c) Not a form of social exclusion and it attracts no significant health issues
   d) An extreme form of social exclusion and attracts significant health issues

4. Mental ill health amongst older people is often further compounded by:
   a) Aging
   b) Physical co-morbidity
   c) Dementia
   d) Lack of pension planning

5. Abuse is about the misuse of power and is based on the principle of:
   a) Whether harm was caused and intended
   b) Whether harm was not caused but intended
   c) Whether harm was caused rather than whether harm was intended
   d) Whether just neglect was apparent

6. In terms of sexual abuse the most prevalent mental health conditions are?
   a) Post-traumatic stress disorder, schizophrenia, suicide and substance abuse
   b) Post-traumatic stress disorder, depression, personality disorders, suicide and substance abuse
   c) Generalised anxiety disorder, depression, suicide and substance abuse
   d) Post-traumatic stress disorder, depression, suicide and substance abuse

7. Higher incidences of depression and anxiety may have resulted from the experience of being lesbian, gay, bisexual or transgender in:
   a) A largely heterosexist and transphobic society
   b) A largely inclusive society
   c) A largely heterosexist society
   d) A largely transphobic society

8. Spirituality means:
   a) The same thing to everyone
   b) Religion
   c) Different things to different people
   d) Religious practice

Answers

Essential skills and knowledge

1. b	12. d	23. a
2. d	13. d	24. c
3. c	14. b	25. d
4. d	15. c	26. c
5. d	16. c	27. a
6. c	17. d	28. c
7. a	18. a	29. c
8. b	19. a	30. b
9. b	20. c	31. c
10. e	21. b	32. a
11. c	22. d	33. b

Conditions

1. b	8. b	15. a
2. d	9. a	16. b
3. b	10. c	17. c
4. d	11. b	18. a
5. a	12. d	19. b
6. c	13. d	
7. c	14. c	

Specific issues

1. b	4. b	7. a
2. a	5. c	8. c
3. d	6. d	

Glossary

Abstinence Supporting an individual to refrain from using a drug and/or alcohol.

Acute detoxification Supporting an individual to withdraw rapidly from an addictive substance.

Adjustment disorders When an individual finds it difficult to adjust or cope with an identifiable life event.

Administrating medication Administering a prescribed medication.

Amenorrhoea The absence of menstrual periods.

Apathy Lack of interest, emotion or concern.

Art therapy Using art as a therapy to deal with difficult emotions in a healthy way.

Assessment Establishing an understanding of a service user's situation through a process of asking questions.

Assessment methods These include using checklists, questionnaires, rating scales, tools, structured interviews, day-to-day observations and interactions.

Authoritarian team leader Autocratic.

Autonomy The ability and freedom to self-govern.

Balanced diet Eating the right amounts of the food groups.

Behavioural activation Utilising reinforcement to influence the development of desired behaviours.

Behavioural therapy A range of behavioural techniques that focus on reinforcing desired behaviours.

Biofeedback A therapeutic approach whereby a person controls their body's functions by receiving physiological information such as controlling heart rate.

Blood pressure The measure of the force of blood or pressure against the vessel walls.

Body mass index (BMI) Bodyweight.

Bradycardia Slow heart rate.

Cannabis A drug that can have a relaxing effect but can also induce confusion, hallucinations, anxiety and paranoia.

Care programme approach (CPA) A risk-management process used within the field of mental health.

Case studies A descriptive exploration of an individual's circumstances.

Rapid Mental Health Nursing, First Edition. Grahame Smith and Rebecca Rylance.
© 2016 John Wiley & Sons, Ltd. Published 2016 by John Wiley & Sons, Ltd.

Catatonic   A disorder of motor function whereby individuals may be still for long periods of time.

Classification   Identifying, grouping and ordering mental disorders.

Clinical governance   A process whereby healthcare organisations improve the quality of the services they provide.

Clinical observations   Temperature, pulse, respiratory rate and blood pressure (also known as vital signs).

Code of conduct   A professional code which nurses are required to adhere to.

Cognitive restructuring   Identifying and changing irrational thoughts.

Cognitive stimulation   A brief psychological treatment for individuals diagnosed with mild to moderate dementia that focuses on providing structured activities that are cognitively stimulating.

Collaboration   Working together within the therapeutic relationship.

Communication   A two-way process that requires the effective use of verbal and non-verbal communication skills.

Coping strategy work   An individual is supported to develop healthy coping strategies.

Creutzfeldt–Jakob disease   A degenerative and fatal disorder of the brain that is progressive and quickly leads to dementia.

Delusion   A fixed, false belief.

Desensitisation   A process of reducing sensitivity by repeated and supported exposure to a difficult situation or stimulus.

Diagnosis   An assessment process that focuses on collecting information and formulating a treatment plan.

Dialectic behaviour therapy   Supporting individuals diagnosed with a borderline personality disorder to cope with emotional difficulties in a healthy way.

Documentation   Record-keeping.

Domains   The required knowledge, skills and attitudes a student nurse needs to attain to qualify. These include professional values; communication and interpersonal skills; nursing practice and decision-making; and leadership, management and team working.

Electroencephalography (EEG)   Measuring the electrical activity of the brain.

Elimination   Bowel and bladder habits.

Empathetic   Being an active listener, genuinely interested, accepting the person and being caring and compassionate.

Empathy   Being able to identify with the service user's experiences.

Encopresis   Voluntary or involuntary soiling.

Enuresis   Inability to control urination usually at night time.

Ethical practice   Utilising the relevant ethical theories, understanding the relevant professional rules and also having the skills to reason ethically.

Ethical reasoning   A systematic process underpinned by an ethical framework.

Ethical theories   Theories that focus on what actions are right, what ought to be done, what motives are good and what characteristics are virtuous.

Ethnography   A research method that focuses on studying and exploring cultural living.

Family therapy   A therapy that focusing on working with families and couples.

Field skills   The knowledge, skills and attitudes that nurses must acquire in order to practise in a specific field of nursing.

Fields of nursing   Formerly known as branches of nursing, there are four fields: mental health, adult, child and development disability.

Focus groups   A research method that explores the opinions, beliefs and attitudes of a group of individuals.

Generic skills   The knowledge, skills and attitudes required of all nurses by the end of a pre-registration nursing programme.

Grade exposure and response prevention   Supporting an individual to confront their obsessions in a structured way.

Grounded theory   The discovery of theory through the research process.

Group therapy   Psychological therapies within a group setting.

Guided self-help   A problem-focused approach that assists individuals to change the way they think, feel and behave.

Hallucination   A perception of the outside world that is perceived as being true even though there is no presence of an external stimulus; for example, hearing a voice when no one is there.

Hallucinogens   A group of drugs that disrupt an individual's sense of reality.

Harm-reduction strategies   Supporting an individual to learn practical strategies that reduce the harms associated with drug use.

Health promotion   Enabling individuals to control and improve their health and well-being.

Huntington's disease   A degenerative and genetic disorder of the brain that is characterised by loss of muscle coordination, and cognitive and mental-health difficulties.

Hyperkinetic disorders   A behavioural syndrome usually seen in children whereby the individual is hyperactive, impulsive and finds it difficult to concentrate.

Hypoglycaemia   Low blood sugar.

Hypothermia   A temperature below 35.0°C.

Incontinence   An inability to control the function of the bladder or bowel.

Infection-control skills   Effective infection prevention and control practices and techniques.

Infection control and prevention   A zero tolerance of infection.

Interpersonal therapy   A time-limited psychological therapy that supports an individual to control their mood and emotions healthily and within the context of their everyday relationships.

Medication adherence   Taking medication as prescribed.

Mental distress   Metal health problems that cannot be fully captured by using the term mental illness.

Mental health nursing practice tree   An illustrative guide to making reasoned decisions for the mental health nurse.

Mentalisation-based approaches   Supporting individuals diagnosed with a borderline personality disorder to recognise and understand the relationship between their actions and their mental states.

Mindfulness approaches   Supporting the individual to focus their attention and awareness.

Motivational enhancement therapy   Supporting individuals to engage in treatment for their drug and/or alcohol use.

Motivational interviewing   A psychological approach that focuses on supporting the individual to change specific behaviours.

Narrative studies   Systematically studying the effective elements of service user's stories.

Neuropsychiatry   A subspeciality of psychiatry that involves both neurology and psychiatry, and deals with mental disorders attributable to diseases of the nervous system.

Normal temperature   A body temperature between 36.0–37.2°C.

Nutritional support   Assisting the service user to meet their nutritional needs.

Opiates   A class of drugs that depress the central nervous system.

Paradoxical intention   A therapy that supports a person to challenge their anxiety through intensifying the anxiety and then working rationally through the emotional state.

Parkinson's disease   A degenerative disorder of the nervous system characterised by movement problems.

Personality   An individual's thinking, feeling and behaving patterns which are viewed either as unique to the individual or as measurable through identifying personality traits.

Pharmacological treatments   Drug treatments.

Phenomenology   The study of an individual's conscious understanding of a given experience.

Pick's Disease   A degenerative disorder of the brain that is characterised by speech, cognitive and behavioural difficulties.

Pink therapy   A talking therapy which focuses on working supportively and positively with gay, lesbian and bisexual people.

Positive risk management   A risk-management approach that is collaborative and recovery focused.

Pre-therapy work   Helping prepare individuals to engage with psychological therapies.

Professional boundaries   Adhering to the Nursing & Midwifery Council's professional code of conduct.

Professional competencies   Competencies that mental health nursing students are professionally required to attain before they qualify.

Psychoeducation   Education about an individual's condition, including how to manage their symptoms.

Psychological interventions   Mental health nursing interventions underpinned by psychological methods and theory with the intention of improving biopsychosocial functioning.

Psychosocial interventions   A type of psychological interventions.

Pulse   The measurement of an individual's heart rate.

Pyrexia   A body temperature above 37.5°C.

Reality orientation therapy   A therapy that focuses on reducing confusion, disorientation and memory loss through orientating the individual to the present time, place and person.

Resilience   An individual's ability to cope with psychosocial adversity.

Respiratory rate   Rate, rhythm and depth of breathing.

Risk   Adverse incidents.

Risk management   A systematic process that focuses on managing identified risk.

Risk management — mental health care   Managing the likelihood that harm to self and/or others will occur.

Social learning strategies   Supporting an individual to learn healthy coping strategies from others (society) that can be used within a social context.

Solution-focused therapy   A brief psychological therapy that is goal oriented and focuses on present and future solutions rather than looking at past problems.

Stimulants   A class of drugs that stimulate the central nervous system.

Stimulation-control therapy   A behavioural approach that links bed with sleep — go to bed when tired.

Strengths model   Focusing on the strengths of the individual and their circumstances to aid recovery.

Stroke   Also known as a cerebrovascular accident, a stroke describes brain function that is adversely affected due to the blood supply being cut off to a part or parts of the brain.

Structured physical activity   Promoting physical activity in a planned way for older adults.

Suicide   Intentional self-inflicted death.

Supportive observations   Levels of observations.

Systemic therapy   A therapy that is concerned with individuals and their relationships and interactions within a group context.

Tachycardia   An abnormally fast resting heart rate.

Therapeutic community treatments   Using a residential group-based approach to treat individuals diagnosed with personality disorders or drug and alcohol problems.

Therapeutic relationship a professional relationship between the mental health nurse and the service user that is partnership focused, person centred and non-discriminatory.

Therapeutic self the nurse being self-aware and use this knowledge in a positive way when working with service users.

The 6C's Communication skills within a nursing context: care, compassion, competence, communication, courage and commitment.

Validation therapy A psychological approach that focuses on respecting the person through the use of structured communication.

Values-based practice a process focusing on managing ethical conflict within the field of mental health practice.

Vascular dementia Dementia caused by vascular problems which can result in the individual having a series of mini-strokes that adversely affect brain function.

Volition Desire or will.

References, further reading and useful resources

References and further reading

Abdel-Khalek, A.M. (2011) Religiosity, subjective well-being, self-esteem, and anxiety among Kuwaiti Muslim adolescents. *Mental Health, Religion and Culture*, **14**(**2**), 129–140.

Adams, T.B., Bezner, J.R., Drabbs, M.E. *et al.* (2000) Conceptualization and measurement of the spiritual and psychological dimensions of wellness in a college population. *Journal of the American College of Health*, **48**(**4**), 165–173.

Adults with Incapacity Act 2000 [WWW document]. URL http://www.legislation.gov.uk/asp/2000/4/contents [accessed on 16 November 2015].

Agrawal, N., Fleminger, S., Ring, H. and Deb, S. (2008) Neuropsychiatry in the UK: Planning the service provision for the 21st century. *Psychiatric Bulletin*, **32**: 303–306.

Aneurin Bevan Health Board (2010) *Guidelines for the treatment of under nutrition in the community including advice on oral nutritional supplement (sip feed) prescribing*. Aneurin Bevan Health Board, Pontypool, UK.

APA (2013). *Classification and Statistical Manual of Mental Disorders (5th Edition)* [WWW document] URL http://www.dsm5.org/pages/default.aspx [accessed on 16 November 2015] American Psychiatric Association, Arlington, VA.

Bach, S. and Ellis, P. (2011) *Leadership, Management and Team Working in Nursing*. Learning Matters, Exeter, UK.

Baker, P. and Cruickshank, J. (2009). I am happy in my faith: the influence of religious affiliation, saliency, and practice on depressive symptoms and treatment preference. *Mental Health, Religion and Culture*, **12**(**4**), 339–357.

Banning M (2008) A review of clinical decision making: models and current research. *Journal of Clinical Nursing*, **17**: 187–195.

Barber, P. (2013) *Medicine Management for Nurses: Case Book*. Open University Press, Maidenhead, UK.

Barber, P. and Robertson, D (2015) *Essentials of Pharmacology for Nurses (3rd Edition)*. Open University Press, Maidenhead, UK.

Baker, P. (ed) (2009) *Psychiatric and Mental Health Nursing: The craft of caring (2nd Edition)*. Hodder Arnold, London.

Barker, P.J. and Buchanan-Barker, P. (2005) *The Tidal Model: A Guide for Mental Health Professionals*. Brunner-Routledge, London.

Rapid Mental Health Nursing, First Edition. Grahame Smith and Rebecca Rylance.
© 2016 John Wiley & Sons, Ltd. Published 2016 by John Wiley & Sons, Ltd.

Benner, P. (1982) From novice to expert. *The American Journal of Nursing*, **82**(**3**), 402–407.

Bortolotti, B., Menchetti, M., Bellini, F. *et al*. (2008) Psychological interventions for major depression in primary care: a meta-analytic review of randomized controlled trials *General Hospital Psychiatry*, **30**(**4**): 293–302.

Boulanger C. and Toghill M (2009) How to measure and record vital signs to ensure detection of deteriorating patients. *Nursing Times*, **105**(**47**): 10–12.

Bowers, L. (2010) How expert nurses communicate with acutely psychotic patients. *Mental Health Practice*, **13**(**7**): 24–26.

Bracken, P. and Thomas, P. (2005) *Postpsychiatry: mental health in a postmodern world*. Oxford University Press, Oxford, UK.

Burton, N. (2006) *Psychiatry*. Blackwell Publishing, Oxford, UK.

Callaghan, P., Playle, J. and Cooper, L. (eds) (2009) *Mental Health Nursing Skills*. Oxford University Press, Oxford, UK.

Care Act 2014 [WWW document]. URL http://www.legislation.gov.uk/ukpga/2014/23/contents/enacted/data.htm [accessed on 16 November 2015].

Carney, G. and Smith, G. (2012) Psychological interventions in psychosis. In Smith, G. (ed) *Psychological Interventions in Mental Health Nursing*. Open University Press, Maidenhead.

Carper, B.A. (1978) Fundamental patterns of knowing in nursing, *Advances in Nursing Science*, **1**(**1**), 13–23.

Castledine, G (2006) The importance of measuring and recording vital signs correctly. *British Journal of Nursing*, **15**(**5**): 285.

Castonguay, L.G. and Oltmans, T.F. (eds) (2013) *Psychopathology: From science to Clinical Practice*. Guildford Press, London.

CBCNO and DoH CAN (2012) *Compassion in Practice*. Commissioning Board Chief Nursing Officer and Department of Health Chief Nursing Adviser, London.

Copeland, M.E. (1997) *Wellness Recovery Action Plan*. Peach Press, Dummerston, VT.

CPAA (2008) *The CPA and Care Standards Handbook (3rd edn.)* Care Programme Approach Association, Chesterfield, UK.

Crook, J.A. (2001) How do expert nurses make on-the-spot clinical decisions? A review of the literature. *Journal of Psychiatric and Mental Health Nursing*, **8**: 1–5.

Crowe, M., Whitehead, L., Wilson, L. *et al*. (2010) Disorder-specific psychosocial interventions for bipolar disorder: A systematic review of the evidence for mental health nursing practice. *International Journal of Nursing Studies*. **47**: 896–908.

Curran, J. and Rogers, P. (2004) Acute psychiatric in-patient assessment. In Harrison, M., Howard, D. and Mitchell, D. (eds) (2004) *Acute Mental Health Nursing: From Acute Concerns to the Capable Practitioner*. Sage, London.

Dahlqvist Jönsson, P., Skärsäter, I., Wijk, H. and Danielson, E. (2011) Experience of living with a family member with bipolar disorder. *International Journal of Mental Health Nursing*, **20**: 29–37.

Davey, G. (2014) *Psychopathology: Research, Assessment and Treatment in Clinical Psychology (2nd Edition)*. Wiley–Blackwell, Oxford.

DoH (2000) *No Secrets. Guidance on developing and implementing multiagency policies and procedures to protect vulnerable adults from abuse.* Department of Health, The Stationery Office, London.

DoH (2004) *The Ten Essential Shared Capabilities: A Framework for the Whole of the Mental Health Workforce.* Department of Health, The Stationery Office, London.

DoH (2006) *From Values to Action: The Chief Nursing Officer's Review of Mental Health Nursing.* Department of Health, The Stationery Office, London.

DoH (2007) *Best Practice in Managing Risk: Principles and Evidence for Best Practice in the Assessment and Management of Risk to Self and Others in Mental Health Services.* Department of Health, The Stationery Office, London.

DoH (2007a) *Briefing 9. Mental health issues within lesbian, gay and bisexual (LGB) communities.* Department of Health, The Stationery Office, London.

DoH (2007b) *Safe, Sensible and Social. The next steps in the National Alcohol Strategy.* Department of Health, The Stationery Office, London.

DoH (2009) *Living Well with Dementia: A National Dementia Strategy.* Department of Health. The Stationery Office, London.

DoH (2009a) *Valuing People Now: A New Three Year Strategy for People with Learning Disabilities.* Department of Health. The Stationery Office, London.

DoH (2010) *Front Line Care: the future of nursing and midwifery in England. Report of the Prime Minister's Commission on the Future of Nursing and Midwifery in England 2010.* Department of Health, The Stationery Office, London.

DoH (2010a) *Nothing Ventured, Nothing Gained: Risk Guidance for People with Dementia.* Department of Health, The Stationery Office, London.

DoH (2011a) *No Health Without Mental Health: A Cross-Government Mental Health Outcomes Strategy for People of All Ages.* Department of Health, The Stationery Office, London.

DoH (2011b) *Talking Therapies: A Four-year Plan of Action: A Supporting Document to No Health Without Mental Health: A Cross-government Mental Health Outcomes Strategy for People of All Ages.* Department of Health, The Stationery Office, London.

DoH (2012) *Vision and Strategy: An Approach to the Nursing and Midwifery Contribution of 'No Health Without Mental Health.* Department of Health, The Stationery Office, London.

DoH (2013) *Patients First and Foremost: The Initial Government Response to the Report of The Mid Staffordshire NHS Foundation Trust Public inquiry.* Department of Health, The Stationery Office, London.

DoH (2015). *Prime Minister's challenge on dementia 2020.* Department of Health, The Stationery Office, London.

Dougherty, L. and Lister, S. (eds) (2011) *The Royal Marsden Hospital Manual of Clinical Nursing Procedures: Student Edition (8th Edition).* Wiley–Blackwell, Chichester, UK.

Downs, M. and Bowers, B. (eds) (2014) *Excellence in Dementia Care (2nd Edition).* Open University Press, Maidenhead, UK.

Enduring Powers of Attorney Order 1987 [WWW document]. URL http://www.legislation.gov.uk/nisi/1987/1627/contents/made [accessed on 16 November 2015].

European Convention on Human Rights 2010 [WWW document]. URL http://www.echr.coe.int/documents/convention_eng.pdf [accessed on 16 November 2015].

Equality Act 2010 [WWW document]. URL http://www.legislation.gov.uk/ukpga/2010/15/contents [accessed on 16 November 2015].

Fox, A.P., Larkin, M. and Leung, N. (2011) The personal meaning of eating disorder symptoms: an interpretative phenomenological analysis. *Journal of Health Psychology*, **16**: 116–125.

Franks, V. (2004) Evidence-based uncertainty in mental health nursing. *Journal of Psychiatric and Mental Health Nursing*, **11**: 99–105.

Geddes, J., Price, J., McKnight, R. (2012) *Psychiatry (4th Edition)*. Oxford University Press, Oxford, UK.

Goldberg, S.E., Whittamore, K.H., Harwood, R.H. *et al.* (2012) The prevalence of mental health problems among older adults admitted as an emergency to a general hospital. *Age and Ageing*, **41**: 80–86.

Goleman, D. "What Makes a Leader?" In Henry, J. (ed) (2007) *Creative Management Development (3rd edition)*. Sage, London.

Gournay, K. (2009) Psychosocial interventions. In R. Newell and K. Gournay (eds) (2009) *Mental Health Nursing: an Evidence-based Approach (2nd edition)*. Churchill Livingstone, London.

Grant, A., Mills, J., Mulhern, R. and Short, N. (2004) The therapeutic alliance and case formulation. In Grant, A., Mills, J., Mulhern, R. and Short, N. (2004) *Cognitive Behavioural Therapy in Mental Health Care*. Sage, London.

Guldin, M.B., Vedsted, P., Jensen, A.B. *et al.* (2013) Bereavement care in general practice: a cluster randomized clinical trial. *Family Practice* **30**, 134–141.

Harris, N., Baker, J. and Gray, R. (eds) (2009) *Medicines Management in Mental Health Care*. Wiley–Blackwell, Chichester, UK.

Hargie, O. (2006) *The Handbook of Communication Skills*. Routledge, Hove, UK.

HMG (2015) *Working together to safeguard children. A guide to inter-agency working to safeguard and promote the welfare of children*. [WWW document]. URL https://www.gov.uk/government/uploads/system/uploads/attachment_data/file/419595/working_together_to_safeguard_children.pdf [accessed 16 November 2015] Her Majesty's Government, London.

Hughes, J., Blackman, H. and McDonald, E., *et al.* (2011) Involving service users in infection control practice. *Nursing Times*; **107**: 25.

Hunot, V., Churchill, R., Teixeira, V. and Silva de Lima, M. (2007) Psychological therapies for generalised anxiety disorder. *Cochrane Database of Systematic Reviews*, Issue 1. Art. No.: CD001848. DOI: 10.1002/14651858.CD001848. pub4.

Human Rights Act 1998 [WWW document]. URL http://www.legislation.gov.uk/ukpga/1998/42/contents [accessed on 16 November 2015].

James, P.D. and Cowman, S. (2007) Psychiatric nurses' knowledge, experience and attitudes towards clients with borderline personality disorder. *Journal of Psychiatric and Mental Health 67Nursing*, **14(7)**: 670–678.

Jasper, M. and Rolfe, G. (2011) Critical reflection and the emergence of professional knowledge. In G. Rolfe, M. Jasper and D. Freshwater (eds) (2011) *Critical Reflection in Practice: Generating Knowledge for Care (2nd edition)*. Palgrave Macmillan, Basingstoke,UK.

Jones, R. (2015) *Mental Health Act Manual (18th Edition)*. Sweet and Maxwell, Basingstoke, UK.

Johnstone, C. and Farley, A. (2006) Nurses' role in nutritional assessment and screening - Part one of a two-part series. *Nursing Times*, **102(49)**: 28.

Katona, C., Cooper, C. and Robertson, M. (2012) *Psychiatry at a Glance (5th Edition)*. Wiley–Blackwell, Oxford, UK.

Kedge, S. and Appleby, B. (2009) Promoting a culture of curiosity within nursing practice. *British Journal of Nursing*, **18(10)**, 635–637.

King, M., Semlyen, J., Tai, S.S. *et al.* (2008) A systematic review of mental disorder, suicide and deliberate self-harm in lesbian, gay and bisexual people. *BMC Psychiatry* **8(1)**, 70.

Lapierre, S., Erlangsen, A., Waern, M. *et al.* (2011) Systematic review of elderly suicide prevention programs. *Crisis*, **32(2)**: 88–98.

Livesley, W.J. (2005) Principles and strategies for treating personality disorder. *Canadian Journal of Psychiatry*, **50(8)**: 442–450.

Lovejoy, M. (1984) Recovery from schizophrenia: a personal odyssey. *Hospital and Community Psychiatry*, **35**: 809–812.

Lovell, K. and Richards, D. (2008) *A Recovery Programme for Depression*. Rethink, London.

Mackeith, J. and Burns, S. (2008) *Mental Health Recovery Star: User Guide*. Mental Health Providers Forum, London.

McKenzie C, Manley K (2011) Leadership and responsive care: Principle of Nursing Practice H. *Nursing Standard*, **25(35)**: 35–37.

McManus, S., Meltzer, H. and Brugha, T. (2009) *Adult Psychiatric Morbidity in England, 2007: Results of a Household Survey*. NHS Information Centre for Health and Social Care, Leeds, UK.

Melvin, P. (2004) A nursing service for homeless people with mental health problems. *Mental Health Practice*. **7(8)**, 28–30.

Mental Capacity Act 2005 [WWW document]. URL www.legislation.gov.uk/ukpga/2005/9/contents [accessed on 16 November 2015].

Mental Health Act 1983 (amended 2007) [WWW document]. URL http://www.legislation.gov.uk/ukpga/2007/12/contents [accessed on 16 November 2015].

Mental Health (Care and Treatment) (Scotland) Act 2003 [WWW document]. URL http://www.legislation.gov.uk/asp/2003/13/contents [accessed on 16 November 2015].

Mental Health Order 1986 [WWW document]. URL http://www.nidirect.gov.uk/the-mental-health-act [accessed on 16 November 2015].

MHF (2007) *Making Space for Spirituality*. [WWW document]. URL http://www.mentalhealth.org.uk/content/assets/PDF/publications/making_space.pdf?view=Standard [accessed on 16 November 2015] Mental Health Foundation, London.

Miller, W.R. and Rollnick, S. (1991) *Motivational Interviewing: Preparing People to Change Addictive Behaviour*. Guildford Press, London.

Mind (2009) *Improving mental health support for refugee communities — an advocacy approach*. [WWW document]. URL http://www.mind.org.uk/media/192447/Refugee_Report_1.pdf [accessed on 16 November 2015] Mind, London.

Moniz-Cook, E. and Manthorpe, J. (eds) (2009) *Early Psychological Interventions in Dementia: Evidence-Based Practice*. Jessica Kingsley, London.

Morrison, J. (2014) *DSM-5 Made Easy: The Clinicians Guide to Diagnosis*. Guildford Press, London.

Mullen, P.E., Martin, J.L., Anderson, J.C. *et al.* (1993) Childhood sexual abuse and mental health in later life. *British Journal of Psychiatry* **163**, 721–732.

Nash, M. (2014) *Physical Health and Well-Being in Mental Health Nursing: Clinical Skills for Practice*. Open University Press, Maidenhead, UK.

NEF (2008) *Five Ways to Well-being: The Evidence*. New Economics Foundation, London.

NHS QIS (2010) *Vital Systems, Supporting Healthcare Improvement in Scotland – Person-centred Safe and Effective Care: Clinical Governance and Risk Management a National Overview*. National Health Service Quality Improvement Scotland, Edinburgh.

NICE (2004) *Guidance on the use of electroconvulsive therapy* – TA59. National Institute for Health and Care Excellence, London.

NICE (2004a) *Eating Disorders: Core Interventions in the Treatment and Management of Anorexia Nervosa, Bulimia Nervosa and Related Eating Disorders – Clinical Guideline 9*. National Institute of Health and Care Excellence, London.

NICE (2004b) *Self-harm: The short-term physical and psychological management and secondary prevention of self-harm in primary and secondary care – Clinical Guideline 16*. National Institute of Health and Care Excellence, London.

NICE (2005) *Depression in Children and Young People: Identification and Management in Primary, Community and Secondary Care – Clinical Guideline 28*. National Institute of Health and Care Excellence, London.

NICE (2005a) *Obsessive-compulsive Disorder: Core Interventions in the Treatment of Obsessive-compulsive Disorder and Body Dysmorphic Disorder*. British Psychological Society and Royal College of Psychiatrists, London.

NICE (2006) *Nutrition support in adults: Oral nutrition support, enteral tube feeding and parenteral nutrition – Clinical Guideline 32*. National Institute for Health and Care Excellence, London.

NICE (2006a) *Bipolar Disorder: The Management of Bipolar Disorder in Adults, Children and Adolescents, in Primary and Secondary Care – Clinical Guideline 38*. National Institute of Health and Care Excellence, London.

NICE (2007) *Faecal Incontinence: The Management of Faecal Incontinence in Adults – Clinical Guideline 49*. National Institute of Health and Care Excellence, London.

NICE (2007a) *Drug Misuse Psychosocial Interventions – NICE Clinical Guideline 51*. National Institute of Health and Care Excellence, London.

NICE (2008) *Attention Deficit Hyperactivity Disorder: Diagnosis and Management of ADHD in Children, Young People and Adults – Clinical Guideline 72*. National Institute of Health and Care Excellence, London.

NICE (2009) *Schizophrenia: Core Interventions in the Treatment and Management of Schizophrenia in Adults in Primary and Secondary Care*. National Institute for Health and Care Excellence, London.

NICE (2009a) *The Treatment and Management of Depression in Adults*. British Psychological Society and Royal College of Psychiatrists, London.

NICE (2011) *Commissioning Stepped Care for People with Common Mental Health Disorders: Clinical Commissioning Guide 41*. National Institute for Health and Care Excellence, London.

NICE (2011a) *Generalised Anxiety Disorder and Panic Disorder (With or Without Agoraphobia) in Adults: Management in Primary, Secondary and*

Community Care. British Psychological Society and Royal College of Psychiatrists, London.

NICE (2011b) *Alcohol-use Disorders, Diagnosis, Assessment and Management of Harmful Drinking and Alcohol Dependence – NICE Clinical Guideline 115*. National Institute of Health and Care Excellence, London.

NICE (2012) *Infection: Prevention and control of healthcare-associated infections in primary and community care – NICE Clinical Guideline 10*. National Institute of Health and Care Excellence, London.

NICE (2014) *Psychosis and schizophrenia in adults: prevention and management*. National Institute for Health and Care Excellence, London.

NICE (2014a) *Self-harm: longer-term management –Clinical Guideline 133*. National Institute of Health and Care Excellence, London.

NICE (2015) *Violence and aggression: short-term management in mental health, health and community settings - Clinical Guideline 39*. National Institute of Health and Care Excellence, London.

NICE–SCIE (2006) *Dementia: Supporting People with Dementia and their Carers in Health and Social Care – NICE Clinical Guideline 42*. National Institute of Health and Care Excellence and Social Care Institute for Excellence, London.

NIHME (2003) *Personality Disorder: No Longer a Diagnosis of Exclusion. Policy Implementation Guidance for the Development of Services for People with Personality Disorder*. National Institute for Mental Health in England, London.

NIPEC (2010) *Evidencing Care: Improving Record Keeping Practice a Guide on Care Planning*. Northern Ireland Practice and Education Council, Belfast.

NMC (2008) *Standards for medicines management*. Nursing & Midwifery Council, London.

NMC (2009) *Record keeping: Guidance for nurses and midwives*. Nursing & Midwifery Council, London.

NMC (2010) *Standards for pre-registration nursing education*. Nursing & Midwifery Council, London.

NMC (2011) *The Prep handbook*. Nursing & Midwifery Council. London.

NMC (2014) *Equality Objectives action Plan*. Nursing and Midwifery Council, London.

NMC (2015) *The Code: Professional Standards of practice and behaviour for nurses and midwives*. Nursing & Midwifery Council, London.

Norman, I. and Ryrie, I. (eds) (2013) *The Art and Science of Mental Health Nursing: Principles and Practice (3rd edition)*. Open University Press, Maidenhead.

NPSA (2007) *Healthcare Risk Assessment Made Easy*. National Patient Safety Agency, London.

NSPCC (2015) *Preventing Child sex abuse. Towards a national strategy for England*. National Society for the Prevention of Cruelty to Children, London.

O'Carroll, M. and Park, A. (2007) *Essential Mental Health Nursing Skills*. Mosby, London.

Ottewill, M., Renshaw, M. and Carmody, J. (2006) Using patient and staff stories to improve risk management. *Nursing Times*, **102(8)**: 34.

Pandya, S. (2009) Antipsychotics: uses, actions and prescribing rationale. *Nurse Prescribing*, **7(1)**: 23–27.

Parahoo, K. (2014) *Nursing research: principles, process and issues (3rd edition)*. Palgrave MacMillan, Basingstoke, UK.

Parker, D. (2012). Psychological interventions and working with the older adult. In: Smith, G. (ed) *Psychological Interventions in Mental Health Nursing*. Open University Press, Maidenhead, UK.

Peate, I. and Nair, M. (2013) *Fundamentals of Applied Pathophysiology: An Essential Guide for Nursing and Healthcare Students (2nd edition)*. Wiley–Blackwell, Chichester, UK.

Peplau, H.E. (1952) *Interpersonal relations in nursing*. G. P. Putnam & Sons, New York.

Person, H. (2009) Transition from nursing student to staff nurse: a personal reflection. *Paediatric Nursing*, **21**(**3**): 30–32.

Phelps, A.C., Lauderdale, K.E., Alcorn, S., *et al*. (2012) Addressing spirituality within the care of patients at the end of line: perspectives of patients with advanced cancer, oncologists and oncology nurses. *Journal of Clinical Oncology*, **30**(**20**), 2538–2544.

QNI (2012) *Mental health and homelessness: guidance for practitioners*. [WWW document]. URL http://qni.org.uk/docs/mental_gealth_guidance_print.pdf [accessed on 16 November 2015] The Queen's Nursing Institute, London.

Raghavan, R., Marshall, M., Lockwood, A. and Duggan, L. (2004) Assessing the needs of people with learning disabilities and mental illness: development of the learning disability version of the Cardinal Needs Schedule (LDCNS). *Journal of Intellectual Disability Research*, **48**(**1**): 25–36.

Raghavan, R. and Patel, P. (2005) *Learning Disabilities and Mental Health: A Nursing Perspective*. Blackwell, Oxford, UK.

RCN (2005) *Managing your stress: A guide for nurses*. Royal College of Nursing, London.

RCN (2006) *Improving continence care for patients: The role of the nurse*. Royal College of Nursing, London.

RCN (2008) *Catheter Care: RCN Guidance for Nurses*. Royal College of Nursing, London.

RCN (2012) *Delegating record keeping and countersigning records: Guidance for nursing staff*. Royal College of Nursing, London.

RCN (2012a) *Essential practice for infection prevention and control: Guidance for nursing staff*. Royal College of Nursing, London.

RCP (2009) *Factsheet: Delirium*. Royal College of Psychiatrists Public Education Editorial Board, London.

RCP (2014) *Spirituality and mental health*. [WWW document]. URL http://www.rcpsych.ac.uk/mentalhealthinformation/therapies/spiritualityandmentalhealth.aspx [accessed on 16 November 2015] Royal College of Psychiatrists, London.

Rea, K. and Ridley, J. (2012) Psychological Interventions in Learning Disability and Mental Health. In Smith, G. (ed) *Psychological Interventions in Mental Health Nursing*. Open University Press, Maidenhead, UK.

Refugee Convention 1951 [WWW document]. URL http://www.unhcr.org/pages/49da0e466.html [accessed on 16 November 2015].

Rigby, P. and Alexander, J. (2008) Building positive therapeutic relationships. In Dooher, J. (ed) *Fundamental Aspects of Mental Health Nursing*. Quay Books, London.

Rober, P. (2008) Being there, experiencing and creating space for dialogue: about working with children in family therapy. *Journal of Family Therapy*, **30**: 465–477.

Rusch, N. and Corrigan, P.W. (2002) Motivational interviewing to improve insight and treatment adherence in schizophrenia. *Psychiatric Rehabilitation Journal*, **26**(**1**): 23–32.

Satori, P. (2010) Spirituality 1: should spiritual and religious beliefs be part of patient care? *Nursing Times*, **106**, 28.

Schofield, I. (2008) Delirium: challenges for clinical governance. *Journal of Nursing Management*, **16**: 127–133.

Schon, D. (1983) From technical rationality to reflection-in-action. In Harrison, R., Reeve, F., Hanson, A. and Clarke, J. (eds) *Supporting Lifelong Learning: Perspectives on Learning*. RoutledgeFalmer, London.

Schwartz, S.J., Zamboanga, B.L., Luyckx, K. *et al.* (2013) Identity in emerging adulthood: reviewing the field and looking forward. *Emerging Adulthood*, **1**(**2**), 96–113.

SCIE (2014). *Adult Safeguarding Resource*. [WWW document]. URL http://www.scie.org.uk/publications/elearning/adultsafeguarding/resource/2_study_area_1_0.html [accessed on 16 November 2015] Social Care Institute for Excellence, London.

Shaffer, V.A. and Zikmund-Fisher, B.J. (2013) All stories are not alike: a purpose-, content-, and valence-based taxonomy of patient narratives in decision aids. *Medical Decision Making*, **33**: 4–13.

Siddiqi, N., Young, J., House, A.O. *et al.* (2011) Stop Delirium! A complex intervention to prevent delirium in care homes: a mixed-methods feasibility study. *Age and Ageing*, **40**: 90–98.

Singh, A.P., Greenwood, N., White, S. and Churchill, R. (2007) Ethnicity and the *Mental Health Act 1983. The British Journal of Psychiatry*, **191**(**2**), 99–105.

Smith, G. (2012) Conclusion: psychological interventions and the mental health nurse's future development. In Smith, G. (ed) *Psychological Interventions in Mental Health Nursing*. Open University Press, Maidenhead, UK.

Smith, G (2014) *Mental Health Nursing at a Glance*. Wiley–Blackwell, Chichester, UK.

SNMAC (1999) *Practice guidance: Safe and supportive observation of patients at risk mental health nursing - Addressing acute concerns*. Standing Nursing and Midwifery Advisory Committee, London.

Spataro, J., Mullen, P.E., Burgess, P.M. *et al.* (2004) Impact of child sexual abuse on mental health. Prospective study in males and females. *The British Journal of Psychiatry*, **184**(**5**), 416–421.

Stevens, S. and Pickering, D. (2010) Keeping good nursing records: a guide. *Community Eye Health*, **23**(**74**): 44–45.

Taylor, D., Paton, C. and Kapur, S. (2015) *The Maudsley Prescribing guidelines in Psychiatry (12th edition)*. Wiley–Blackwell, Chichester, UK.

The Children Act 1989, amended 2004 [WWW document]. URL http://www.legislation.gov.uk/ukpga/2004/31 [accessed on 16 November 2015].

Thompson, N. (2009) *People Skills (3rd edition)*. Palgrave Macmillan, Basingstoke, UK.

Waterworth S. (2003) Time management strategies in nursing practice. *Journal of Advanced Nursing*, **43**(**5**): 432–440.

Watson, D. (2006) The impact of accurate patient assessment on quality of care. *Nursing Times*, **102**(**6**): 34–37.

Welsh, I. and Lyons, C.M. (2001) Evidence-based care and the case for intuition and tacit knowledge in clinical assessment and decision making in mental health nursing practice: an empirical contribution to the debate. *Journal of Psychiatric and Mental Health Nursing*, **8**: 299–305.

WHO (2010). Chapter V: Mental and behavioural disorders In: WHO, *International Classification of Diseases*. [WWW document]. URL http://apps. who.int/classifications/icd10/browse/2016/en#/V [accessed on 16 November 2015] World Health Organization, Geneva.

Wilson, K., Mottram, P.G. and Vassilas, C. (2008) Psychotherapeutic treatments for older depressed people, Cochrane Database of Systematic Reviews, issue **1**.

Woodbridge, K. and Fulford, K.W.M. (2004) *Whose Values? A Workbook for Values-based Practice in Mental Health Care*. Sainsbury Centre for Mental Health, London.

Wright, K.M. (2010) Therapeutic relationship: Developing a new understanding for nurses and care workers within an eating disorder unit. *International Journal of Mental Health Nursing*, **19**: 154–161.

Wright, P. (2006) *Core Psychopharmacology*. Saunders Elsevier, London.

Useful resources

A Guide to the *Mental Health Act 1983 (amended 2007)*
   http://www.mind.org.uk/information-support/legal-rights/mental-health-act/
A Guide to the *Mental Health (Care and Treatment) (Scotland) Act 2003*
   http://www.mwcscot.org.uk/the-law/mental-health-act/
Alzheimer's Society
   http://www.alzheimers.org.uk/
Anatomy and physiology
   http://www.cartercenter.org/documents/ethiopia_health/lecture/plain/nurse/
   LN_human_anat_final.pdf
British National Formulary
   http://www.bnf.org/bnf/index.htm
Care Quality Commission
   http://www.cqc.org.uk/
Dementia UK
   http://www.dementiauk.org/
Department of Health
   https://www.gov.uk/government/organisations/department-of-health
Diagnostic and Statistical Manual of Mental Disorders (DSM-5)
   http://www.dsm5.org/Pages/Default.aspx
Electroconvulsive therapy
   http://www.mind.org.uk/information-support/drugs-and-treatments/
   electroconvulsive-therapy-ect/
Electroconvulsive therapy advice
   http://www.rcpsych.ac.uk/expertadvice/treatmentswellbeing/ect.aspx
Institute of Medical Ethics
   http://instituteofmedicalethics.org/website/
International Classification of Diseases (ICD)
   http://www.who.int/classifications/icd/en/

Medication
   http://www.mind.org.uk/mental_health_a-z/8056_drugs_an_alphabetical_list
Mental Health Foundation
   http://www.mentalhealth.org.uk/
Mental Health Law On-line
   http://www.mentalhealthlaw.co.uk/Main_Page
Mental Health Legislation News
   http://www.mind.org.uk/news?gclid=coca9nnkk7kcfsxltaoddvoaoa
Mind
   http://www.mind.org.uk/
Nursing & Midwifery Council
   http://www.nmc.org.uk/
Nursing Leadership
   http://www.nursingleadership.org.uk/
PACE (LGBT+ mental health charity)
   http://www.pacehealth.org.uk/
Refugee Council
   https://www.refugeecouncil.org.uk/
Rethink Mental Illness
   http://www.rethink.org/
Royal College of Nursing professional development
   http://www.rcn.org.uk/development
Royal College of Psychiatrists
   http://www.rcpsych.ac.uk/usefulresources.aspx
Social Care Institute for Excellence
   http://www.scie.org.uk/
The Foundation of Nursing Leadership
   http://www.nursingleadership.org.uk/
Time management tips
   http://nursingstandard.rcnpublishing.co.uk/students/from-student-to-
   qualified-nurse/effective-time-management-for-nurses
UK Legislation
   http://www.legislation.gov.uk/

Index

Rapid Mental Health Nursing, First Edition. Grahame Smith and Rebecca Rylance.
© 2016 John Wiley & Sons, Ltd. Published 2016 by John Wiley & Sons, Ltd.